VISION IN
VERTEBRATES

VISION IN VERTEBRATES

M. A. Ali
and
M. A. Klyne

Université de Montréal
Montreal, Quebec, Canada

PLENUM PRESS • NEW YORK AND LONDON

Library of Congress Cataloging in Publication Data

Ali, M. A. (Mohamed Ather), 1932–
  Vision in vertebrates.

  Includes bibliographies and indexes.
  1. Vision. 2. Eye. 3. Vertebrates — Physiology. I. Klyne, M. A. II. Title. [DNLM: 1.
Eye — physiology. 2. Vertebrates. 3. Vision. WW 103 A398v]
QP475.A45   1985   596'.01'823   85-12141
ISBN 0-306-42065-1

©1985 Plenum Press, New York
A Division of Plenum Publishing Corporation
233 Spring Street, New York, N.Y. 10013

Printed in the United States of America

PREFACE

When Dr. Katherine Tansley's "Vision in Vertebrates" appeared in 1965, it filled a real void that had hitherto existed. It did so by serving at once as a text-book: for an undergraduate course, a general introduction to the subject for post-graduate students embarking on research on some aspect of vision, and the interested non-specialists. Gordon Walls' "The Vertebrate Eye and Its Adaptive Radiation" and A. Rochon-Duvigneaud's "Les Yeux et la Vision des Vertébrés" have served as important sources of information on the subject and continue to do so even though it is 40 years since they appeared. However, they are essentially specialised reference works and are not easily accessible to boot. The genius of Katherine Tansley was to present in a succinct (132 pages) and lucid way a clear and an interesting survey of the matter. Everyone liked it, particularly the students because one could read it quickly and understand it. Thus, when it seemed that a new edition was desirable, especially in view of the enormous strides made and the vast literature that had accumulated in the past 20 years, one of us (MAA) asked Dr. Tansley if she would undertake the task. Since she is in retirement and her health not in a very satisfactory state both she and her son, John Lythgoe (himself a specialist of vision), asked us to take over the task. In view of the advances made and in view of the fact that it will virtually be impossible anymore to put everything in 100 to 150 pages, we decided to prepare an altogether new book, larger in size, inspiring ourselves however from Dr. Tansley's approach. We have illustrated the book abundantly and attempted to give as many references as possible, obviously putting emphasis on those that are reviews and books. There are a number of specialised works, such as the "Handbook of Sensory Physiology" series that serve particularly the specialist as references. Our aim is to attempt to

v

present the subject in a concise way so that an under-graduate or a beginning graduate student is able to get an overall view of the way vertebrates see. We hope that we have mostly succeeded in doing this. We should welcome comments and criticisms from interested readers.

We thank Madame Hoda Farid for assistance with the preparation of the illustrations, Monsieur Jean-Luc Verville for photographic help and Mademoiselle Francine Chatelois for preparing the index. We appreciate the encouragement we received from our editor, Mr. Kirk Jensen. Preparation of this book was also aided by an operating grant from the Natural Sciences and Engineering Council of Canada.

Montréal, Spring 1985

M. A. Ali
M. A. Klyne

TABLE OF CONTENTS

1

STRUCTURE OF THE VERTEBRATE EYE

The basic pattern of all vertebrate eyes is similar. The cross-section of the eyeball can be represented by a circle with one-fifth of its circumference removed. Into this is fitted a clear segment which has a slightly smaller radius of curvature (cornea). The outer coat, which makes up the remaining four-fifths of the eyeball, is a tough fibrous structure whose opaque posterior part (sclera) is continuous with the strongly curved, transparent cornea (Fig. 1.1). The vertebrate eye may be compared to the camera, and this analogy is illustrated in Fig. 1.2.

In terresterial animals good vision is largely dependent on the optical perfection of the anterior surface of the cornea, and since this surface is exposed it must be well protected. This is done by the lids and by the secretion of tear fluid. The eyelids are composed of compressed fibrous tissue containing muscles and glands. The eyelids close reflexly at the approach of a foreign body, e.g. if the cornea is touched or if the light is too intense. In addition, many animals (e.g. frogs, some birds) have a nictitating membrane or third eyelid composed of transparent and semi-transparent tissues which can be drawn horizontally across the eye between the other two eyelids. Some animals (e.g. snakes) do not have eyelids but possess a 'spectacle' instead - a covering of transparent skin continuous with the skin of the head. Further protection of the cornea is afforded by tear fluid secreted by the lacrimal and Harderian glands. The tear fluid, which varies in composition in different animals, serves to irrigate the anterior surface of the cornea and the inner surface of the eyelids, as well as to wash dust and other foreign particles out of the eye. In some aquatic mammals (e.g. seals) it protects the cornea from salt water.

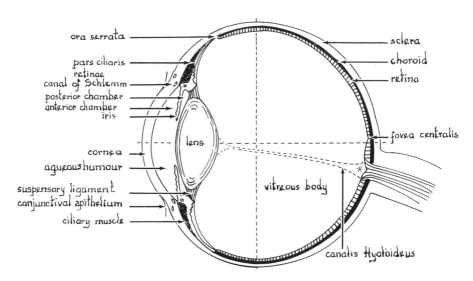

Fig. 1.1: Mid-section through a vertebrate (human) eye illustrating its basic features.
(* - blind spot)

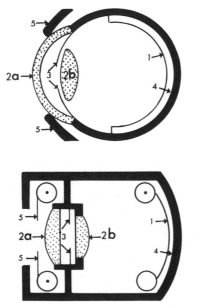

Fig. 1.2: Comparison of eye and camera.

Parts which correspond in function bear similar numbers.

1   -retina = film, on curved track;

2a   -cornea = front element of lens;

2b   -crystalline lens = rear element of lens;

3   -iris = diaphragam be-tween lens elements;

4   -pigment of choroid coat = flat black paint;

5   -eyelids = roller-blind.

(After Walls, 1942)

Light enters the eye through the cornea, passes through the aqueous humour in the anterior chamber, the pupillary aperture of the iris, the lens and the vitreous body before striking the retinal layer that lines the posterior two-thirds of the eyeball (Figs. 1.1, 1.3). The choroid, a vascular pigmented layer which prevents blurring or multiplication of the retinal image by internal reflexions, is a continuation of the iris, and separates the retina from the sclera. Nerve fibres which arise in the retina run across the retinal surface and exit the eyeball through the posterior perforation of the sclera, the optic nerve. These fibres convey the nervous

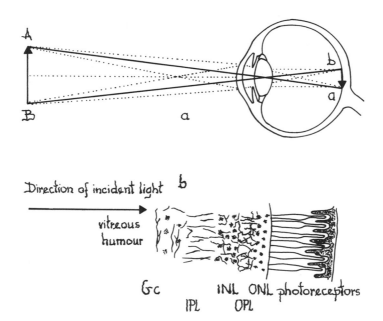

Fig. 1.3a: Formation on the retina of the focussed image **ab** of an object **AB**. The 'optical centre' of the eye is at the cross point of the straight lines **Aa** and **Bb**. This diagrammatic representation is valid only for retinal images close to the axis of the eye.

Fig. 1.3b: Diagram illustrating the path of light through the retina.

GC   -ganglion cell layer;
IPL   -inner plexiform layer;
INL   -inner nuclear layer;
OPL   -outer plexiform layer;
ONL -outer nuclear layer.

impulses, set off by photons striking the retina, to the brain where they give rise to visual sensations.

Cornea

The cornea is the projecting, transparent part of the outermost layer of the eyeball. It is convex anteriorly, and its degree of curvature varies in different individuals and in the same individual during different periods of life.

The cornea consists of four layers. The outermost layer, the conjunctival epithelium, which consists of several strata of epithelial cells covers the cornea proper. The proper substance of the cornea (substantia propria) lies beneath the conjunctival epithelium. It is fibrous, tough, unyielding, perfectly transparent and continuous with the sclera. It consists of flattened lamellae, composed of collagen, superimposed on one another. These lamellae are connected with one another by an interstitial cement substance in which are spaces (corneal spaces). These spaces are stellate in shape and each contains a cell, the corneal corpuscle. Between the conjunctival epithelium and the cornea proper is a layer of closely interwoven fibrils similar to those found in the cornea proper, but without the corneal corpuscles. This layer was named anterior elastic lamina by Bowman and anterior limiting layer by Reichert.

The posterior elastic lamina (membrane of Descemet or Demours) is the posterior-most layer covering the cornea proper. It is an elastic and transparent membrane whose function appears to be the preservation of the requisite permanent correct curvature of the cornea proper. At the margin of the cornea this elastic membrane breaks up into fibres to form a reticular structure at the outer angle of the anterior chamber, the intervals between the fibres forming the spaces of Fontana. These communicate with a circular canal in the sclera (the canal of Schlemm or sinus venosus scleroe) close to its junction with the cornea. The canal of Schlemm communicates internally with the anterior chamber through the spaces of Fontana and externally with the scleral veins. Some of the fibres of this structure are continued into the front of the iris forming the ligamentum pectinatum iridis, while others are connected with the fore part of the sclera and choroid (Fig. 1.4).

The endothelial lining of the aqueous chamber which covers the posterior surface of the elastic lamina is reflected on to the front of the iris and it also lines the spaces of Fontana. This layer consists of a single layer of polygonal, flattened, transparent, nucleated cells.

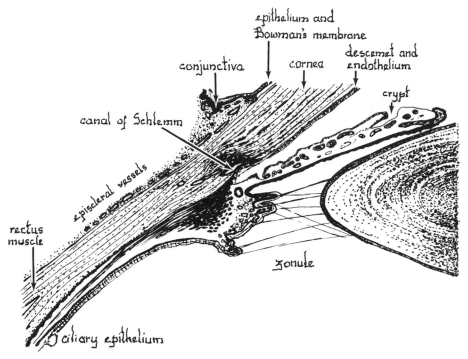

Fig. 1.4: Section of the eye, showing the relationship between the cornea, sclerotic and iris, together with the ciliary muscle and choroid. (After Tansley, 1965)

Aqueous Humour

The aqueous humour is a saline fluid, with an alkaline reaction occupying the anterior chamber and the posterior chamber. This fluid is continuously produced by the epithelial glands of the ciliary body (ciliary glands) and drains out through the canal of Schlemm. The continuous production and flow of the aqueous humour is associated with the existence of a greater pressure within the eyeball than without. Maintenance of this intraocular pressure (10 - 20 mm Hg in man) is important for maintaining the rigidity of the eyeball. However, failure of the aqueous humour to drain, due to the blockage of the drainage channel, leads to higher intraocular pressure and impediment of retinal and choroidal circulation, hence retinal damage (glaucoma).

Iris

The iris is a thin, circular-shaped screen suspended in the aqueous humour behind the cornea, and in front of the lens (Fig. 1.1). The iris is perforated by an aperture, the pupil, for the passage of light. The quantity of light entering the eye in some vertebrates is greatly controlled by the degree of contraction and relaxation of the iris. At its circumference, the iris is continuous with the ciliary body and it is also connected to the posterior elastic lamina of the cornea by means of the pectinate ligament; its inner or free edge forms the margin of the pupil (Fig. 1.4). The surfaces of the iris are flattened; the anterior faces the cornea; and the posterior, the ciliary processes and lens.

The iris is composed of an anterior layer of flattened endothelial cells, the stroma (fibres and cells), and a muscular fibre layer - circular (sphincter pupillae) and radiating (dilator pupillae) fibres - which controls the pupil size. Pigmentation of the iris gives the eye its colour. In the case of blue eyes several layers of small, round or polyhedral cells containing dark pigment are found on the posterior surface of the iris. These cells are continuous with the pigmentary lining of the ciliary process. The colour of the eye is thus due to the degree to which the colouring matter shows through the texture of the iris. In grey, brown and black eyes, pigment granules found in the stroma cells and in the anterior epithelial layer of the iris impart the dark colour to the eye. Completely unpigmented eyes, as found in albinos, appear pink because the blood vessels are then visible.

The size of the aperture (pupil) can be varied in many species by contractile elements in the iris tissue. Some of these are fully developed involuntary muscle fibres which are organised into a ring-shaped sphincter closely surrounding the pupil. Contraction of the sphincter reduces the size of the aperture. In man, the dilator fibres are not proper muscle fibres, but modified tissue elements developed from the anterior face of the retinal part of the iris. However, in birds which have very active pupils both sphincter and dilator are formed of striated muscle fibres and may be under voluntary control. In other species (e.g. teleost fishes) the iris muscles are poorly developed and the pupil is nearly, if not entirely, immobile. Such species have other means of regulating the amount of light reaching the retina (Chapter 6).

The function of the iris is to regulate the amount of light reaching the retina. It therefore shows a reflex contraction of the sphincter, thus decreasing the pupil diameter, in bright light; and a reflex relaxation, with increase in aperture size, when the light is dim. Contraction of the iris also increases the sharpness of the retinal image by preventing light from passing through the less optically perfect lens periphery (Chapter 4). In most species the pupil is circular, however, other forms do occur as modifications to habits and habitats (Chapters 6, 7).

Ciliary Body

The ciliary body is composed of the orbiculus ciliaris, the ciliary processes and the ciliary muscle. The orbiculus ciliaris is directly continuous with the anterior part of the choroid.

The ciliary processes are formed by the plaiting and infolding of the various layers of the choroid at its anterior margin, and are received between corresponding foldings of the suspensory ligament of the lens. They are arranged in a circle, and form a sort of plaited frill behind the iris, around the margin of the lens.

The ciliary muscle consists of a circular band of unstriped fibres on the outer surface of the fore part of the choroid. It consists of two sets of fibres - radiating and circular. The former arise at the point of junction of the cornea and sclera, and partly also from the ligamentum pectinatum iridis; and passing backward are attached to the choroid opposite to the ciliary processes. The circular fibres are internal to the radiating ones and have a circular course around the attachment of the iris. They are well developed in hypermetropic, but are rudimentary or absent in myopic eyes. The ciliary muscle is thought to be the chief agent of accommodation - adjusting the eye to the vision of near objects (Chapter 4).

Crystalline Lens

The crystalline lens, enclosed in the capsule, is situated immediately behind the pupil, in front of the vitreous body, and encircled by the ciliary processes.

The capsule of the lens is a transparent, highly elastic and brittle membrane which closely surrounds the lens. It rests, behind, in the fore part of the vitreous body, in front it is in contact with the free border of the iris, the latter receding from it at the circumference, thus forming the posterior chamber of the eye (Fig. 1.1). It is retained in its position chiefly by the suspensory ligament.

The lens is a transparent, biconvex body; the convexity being greater on the posterior than on the anterior surface. The central points of its anterior and posterior surfaces are called anterior and posterior poles. It consists of concentric layers (substantia corticalis and nucleus lentis), and faint lines radiate from the anterior and posterior poles to the circumference of the lens.

Vitreous Body

The vitreous body forms about four-fifths of the entire globe of the eye. It fills the concavity of the retina, and is hollowed in front forming a deep concavity (the fossa patellaris) for the reception of the lens. It is perfectly transparent, of the consistence of thin jelly, and is composed of an albuminous fluid enclosed in a delicate, transparent membrane - membrana hyaloidea. In the centre of the vitreous, running from the centre of the optic nerve to the posterior surface of the lens is a canal (Canal of Stilling) which is filled with fluid and lined by a prolongation of the hyaloid membrane.

Retina

The retina, an extension of the brain, is a delicate nervous tissue which receives the images of external objects. Its outer surface is in contact with the choroid and its inner surface with the vitreous body. Behind, it is continuous with the optic nerve, and it gradually decreases in thickness from behind forward; and, in front it extends nearly as far as the ciliary body where it appears to terminate in a jagged margin, the ora serrata. Here the nervous tissue of the retina ends, but a thin prolongation of the membrane (pigmentary layer and a layer of columnar epithelium) extends forward over the back of the ciliary processes and iris, forming the pars ciliaris retinae and pars iridica retinae.

The fine structure of the retina is given in Fig. 1.5. The actual photosensitive cells (rods and cones) lie in the outermost layer of the retina next to the pigment epithelium layer - a layer not directly concerned with photoreception. Except in the foveal region, light reaching the photoreceptors must first pass through the other layers of the retina. The fovea is a small depression in the retina formed by lateral displacement of the cells of the inner retinal layers (Fig. 1.6). The fovea centralis is situated near the optic axis of the eye and is responsible for high visual acuity. It is a region of the retina (in a duplex retina) which contains only cones

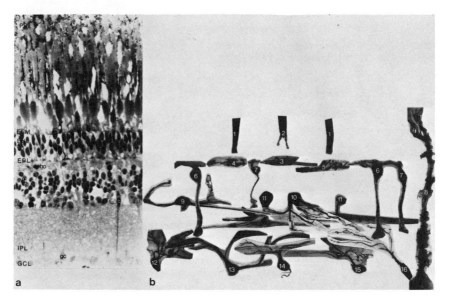

Fig. 1.5:   (a) Transverse section through the retina of
Salvelinus fontinalis. (b) Gives details of the interconnexion
of photoreceptors (1, 2); horizontal cells(3, 4, 5); bipolar cells
(6, 7); amacrine cells (9, 10, 11); and ganglion cells (12 - 16). A
Müller cell (8) is also shown. (From Ali & Wagner, 1980)

and no rods. The cones in this region are different in shape from
cones of the peripherial retina. They are much longer and thinner
such that they somewhat resemble rods (Fig. 1.6).   Another
specialised region of the retina is the optic disc or papilla. It is
that region of the retina where the optic nerve enters the eye. It is
called the blind spot because it is insensitive to light.   The
existence of the blind spot can be easily demonstrated by the
following simple experiment. Closing the left eye, look steadily at
the star in Fig. 1.7. By moving the page slowly towards and away
from the eye a position will be found such that the black disc will
disappear, as its image will then fall entirely on the blind spot of
the right eye.

     Generally, rods and cones are found side by side over most of
the retina, however, variations exist. The rods and cones make
synaptic contact with bipolar cells (outer plexiform layer) and
these in turn contact with the ganglion cells (inner plexiform
layer). The ganglion cells give rise to the optic nerve fibres which

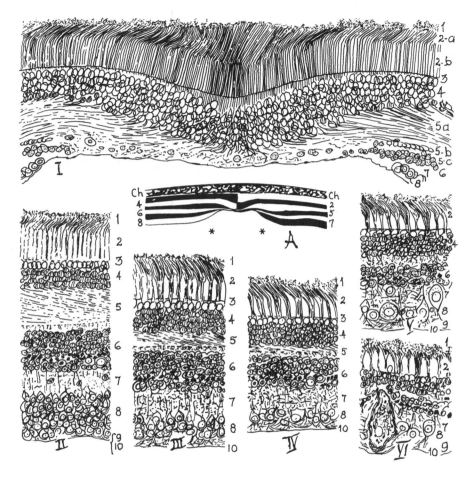

Fig. 1.6: Regional variation of retinal structure in Rhesus
Macaque. **I**, centre of central fovea showing greatly length-
ened, much thinner, and more numerous central cones (slightly
disarrayed), which, together with their nuclei in the fourth
layer, are alone present in the central "rodless area"; at some
distance from the centre, smaller and darker rod nuclei in **4**
begin to appear singly and in groups; lower layers below **4**, in
the centre, are much reduced, fibrous zone **5-a** greatly so,
while zones **5-b** and **5-c** are entirely absent, as are also layers
6-9; **A**, sketch at lower magnification of central fovea and its
immediate vicinity of central area, ** marking the limits of
the foveal pit; note a well-developed choroid membrane, **Ch**;
II, perifoveal region with five tiers of ganglion cells; **III**,
perifoveal region in the periphery of the central area, with

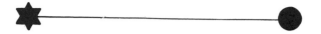

Fig. 1.7: Demonstration of the blind spot. Close the left eye and look steadily at the "star". Move the page towards and away from the observer. At a certain position the black disc will disappear. This corresponds to the blind spot of the right eye.

run towards the optic nerve. Ganglion cells, and to a lesser extent, bipolar cells can have extensively spreading dendrites so that each cell may be influenced by the activity of a large number of rods and cones. Further lateral interactions are mediated by the horizontal and amacrine cells (Fig. 1.5). The retinal structures are held together by a system of supporting (glial) fibres usually known as the radial or Müller fibres. The outer ends of the Müller fibres form a network (outer limiting membrane), and it is through these holes through which the visual cells protrude. The inner ends of the Müller fibres expand into trumpets or pyramids whose bases lie in contact with one another and form an unbroken mosaic (inner limiting membrane) which is the most internal layer of the retina and is in contact with the hyaloid membrane of the vitreous body. There are two nuclear layers in the retina. The outer nuclear layer contains the nuclei of the visual cells (rods and cones) and is situated just internal of the outer limiting membrane. The inner nuclear layer, which contains the nuclei of the horizontal, bipolar and amacrine cells, is located between the outer and inner plexiform layers. Nuclei of the Müller fibres are also found in the inner nuclear layer. The thickness of the nuclear layers reflects to a large extent, retinal adaptations and gives a good indication of the acuity and sensitivity of the retina (Chapters 6, 7).

ganglion cell layer reduced to three tiers; **IV**, near periphery, with ganglion layer represented by a single continuous cell row; **V**, middle periphery with a partly discontinuous layer of much larger ganglion cells; **VI**, far periphery of retina along ora serrata or ora terminalis. (From Polyak, 1968)

Development

The optic nerve and the retina are developed as an outgrowth from the fore brain which extends towards the side of the head. There it is met by an ingrowth from the epiblast from which the lens and epithelium of the conjunctiva and cornea are developed.

The eye is not a secondarily derived appendage of the brain that grows outward to reach the integument, rather the medullary plate and subsequent neural tube are formed from surface ectoderm. The first appearance of the eye is a hollow protrusion of the fore brain, this is called the primitive optic vesicle. It is initially an open cavity then the epiblast lying immediately over it becomes thickened, next a depression, which gradually encroaches on the most prominent part of the primitive ocular vesicle, is formed. This in turn appears to recede before the epiblast so as to become at first depressed and then inverted, thus the cavity of the vesicle is almost obliterated by the folding back of its anterior half. The original vesicle is thus converted into a cap, the optic cap, in which the involuted epiblast, the rudiment of the lens, is received. At the same time the proximal part of the vesicle becomes elongated and narrowed into a hollow stalk, the optic stalk (nerve). Therefore, this cup-shaped cavity consists of two layers:- one, the outer (originally the posterior half of the primitive ocular vesicle) is thin and eventually forms the pigmented layer of the retina; while the other layer, the inner (originally anterior and more prominent part of the ocular vesicle) is much thicker and is converted into the nervous layer of the retina (Fig. 1.8). Thus, as the retina is developed from a protrusion, followed by an invagination, the visual cells lie on the outer retinal surface turned away from the light.

A theory advanced to explain the arrangement of the retina such that the photoreceptors face away from the light source was first proposed by Balfour in 1881 (see Walls, 1942) and elaborated by Polyak (1968). This theory can be further expanded to explain the derivation of the entire optic system (Fig. 1.9):-
a.   An early ancestor had only surface ectoderm. Part of this differentiated into neuroectoderm - similar to the open neural plate stage of human embryonic development. The most superficial cells of the primordial neuroectoderm possessed photoreceptive characteristics for crude differentiation of light intensity. Similar photoreceptors are found in the integument of the earthworm and some other invertebrates.
b.   The evolution of bilateral symmetry as the basic feature of

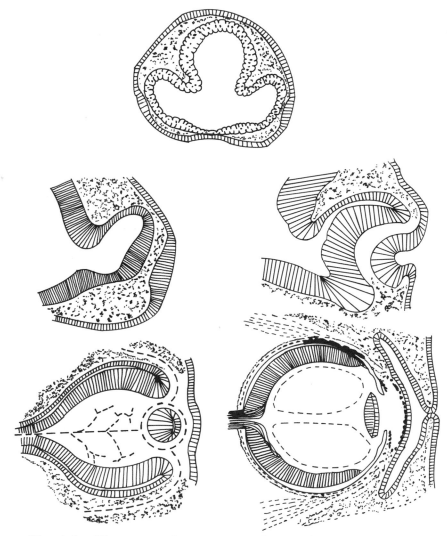

Fig. 1.8: Diagrammatic representation of the development of the vertebrate eye.

the vertebrate body, coupled to an incipient median invagination, saw the concentration of the photoreceptive epithelium into paired placodes. This resulted in more precise localisation of light and shadow. The neuroectodermal cells underlying the photoreceptors differentiated into neurones -

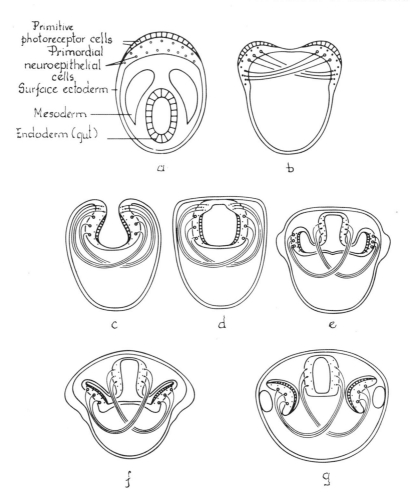

Fig. 1.9: Diagrammatic representation of the evolution of inverted photoreceptors. (See text for details)

some of which developed into bipolar cells and others into ganglion cells. The latter had axons which grew across the midline to innervate motor neurones in the contralateral neuroectoderm of the bilaterally symmetric animal. The crossing axons were the primordial optic nerve fibres. The decussation provided a reflexive pathway for coiling away from the threatened side. Crude differentiation of light intensity was the next probable step in the evolution of vision. However, the actual perception of images had to await the evolution of the optic cup, lens and other structures for image focussing as well as the development of cerebral centres capable of handling complex information.

c.   The entire neural plate, including the optic placodes invaginated.

d.   The closed neural tube is formed. The proposal (Studnicka, 1898) that the retina originated from ciliated ependyma of the third ventricle is probable. Eakin (1962) found ciliary appendages of cells lining the cerebral vesicle (third ventricle) of amphioxus. He suggested that these processes may be light sensitive and demonstrated that the rods and cones of the retina of vertebrates are modified cilia.

e.   Cerebral tissue proliferated in the dorsal region, thus allowing photoreceptor cells to retain proximity to sources of light at the skin. Next, the epidermis overlying the optic vesicles thickened and formed the lens placode.

f., g. The optic vesicle invaginated and the retina was formed as in 'modern' embryos. The continuity of the optic vesicle with the ventricular system of the brain was gradually obliterated. The optic nerves continued to decussate ventral to the neural tube. The glial component of the optic nerve was partly derived from the obliterated stalk of the optic vesicle.

The portion of the wall of the neural tube receiving the decussated optic nerve fibres developed into two structures. The caudal part into the optic tectum (superior colliculus), and the rostral portion into the dorsal thalamus.

Thus the retina and optic centres of the brain were derived from a common neuroectoderm. The optic tectum eventually formed the roof of the midbrain, but in lower vertebrates, in which the cerebral aqueduct is yet unformed, the optic tectum extends over the mid brain as a laminated cortex, continuous at its rostral end with the diencephalon and separated from the underlying midbrain by extensions of the third ventricle (the optic ventricles). Thalamic nuclei also extend into the tegmentum of the mid brain in submammalian vertebrates, examplified by the nucleus rotundus (pulvinar) of reptiles. Optic nerve fibres terminate chiefly in the optic tectum in submammalian vertebrates, but some fibres also end in the thalamus; the termination of these fibres in mammals is proportionately reversed, the majority ending in the thalamus.

Eye Movements

Not all vertebrates exhibit eye movements, but all, except those which have tiny eyes and are virtually blind (such as cave fishes and cave salamanders) have the same six extra ocular muscles. These are arranged in pairs and are :- the superior and inferior recti; the internal and external recti; and the superior and inferior oblique muscles (Fig. 1.10). The superior rectus turns the

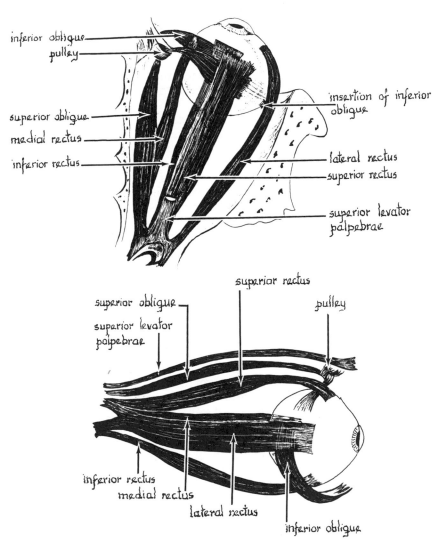

Fig. 1.10: Oculomotor muscles of man as seen from above in a dissected head (a); and laterally (b). In both cases the right eye is shown.

eye upwards and inwards and at the same time rotates the right eye in a clockwise direction and the left eye in a counter-clockwise direction, when viewed from in front. The inferior rectus turns the eye downwards and inwards as well as rotating the right eye counter-clockwise and the left eye clockwise. Contraction of the internal rectus rotates the eye towards the nose while the external rectus rotates the eye outwards. The superior oblique turns the eye down and out, and rotates the right eye clockwise and the left eye counter-clockwise. The inferior oblique turns the eye upwards and outwards, and rotates the right eye counter-clockwise and left eye clockwise.

Eye movements are of two kinds:- voluntary and involuntary. Involuntary eye movements are reflex and autonomic, and their purpose is to keep the visual field as constant as possible during movements of the head and body. Involuntary eye movements are always coordinated - the two eyes always move in the same sense. Voluntary eye movements may or may not be coordinated. Most lizards and all birds (except the owls) are able to move their eyes independently. Mammals (and mammals only) show conjugate eye movements, they are quite incapable of the voluntary moving of one eye independently of the other. Most fish have only involuntary reflex eye movements. Voluntary eye movements are always associated with the presence of fovea or other retinal area of superior vision. Those fishes which possess a fovea are also capable of voluntary convergence on an interesting object in the vicinity. Amphibians are only capable of involuntary reflex movements to retract or elevate the eyes, while reptiles are capable of involuntary eye movements. Independent eye movements reach their highest development in the chameleon which can aim one eye backwards while the other looks forwards. Snakes which have little spontaneous ocular mobility compensate for this by continual side to side movements of the head. Birds have very large eyes which are a tight fit in the orbit and so exhibit very little eye movement, even involuntary. This is replaced by reflex movements of the head. The majority of mammals show little voluntary eye movement, however as they prefer to examine objects binocularly they do so by head movements. In species with lateral eyes, binocular vision is restricted to distant objects; while those with frontal eyes have very good binocular vision.

2

PHYSIOLOGY OF THE RETINA

The vertebrate retina contains specialised cells (photo-receptors) whose function is to absorb light. Generally, two types of photoreceptors are present - rods and cones. Although basically of similar design, these cells are distinguishable morphologically. However, problems may arise when the retina contains only one type of photoreceptor. It may then be necessary to resort to physiological studies before proper identification is possible.

Fundamentally all photoreceptors consist of an outer segment, an inner segment, a nucleus and a synapse (from the sclerad to vitread direction). The outer and inner segments are sclerad of the outer (external) limiting membrane; the nuclei of the photoreceptors form the outer nuclear layer; and the synapses are situated in the outer (external) plexiform layer. The next layer, the innear nuclear layer, contains the nuclei of the secondary neurones (horizontal, bipolar and amacrine cells). These neurones send processes to both the outer (horizontal and bipolar cells) and the inner (bipolar and amacrine cells) plexiform layers. The inner plexiform layer, in addition to receiving processes from bipolar and amacrine cells, also receives processes from ganglion cells. The latter being the final cells through which the light impulse must traverse before leaving the retina (Fig. 2.1).

Photoreceptors

The Outer Segment

The outer segments of the photoreceptor cells are embedded within the apical processes arising from the pigment epithelial

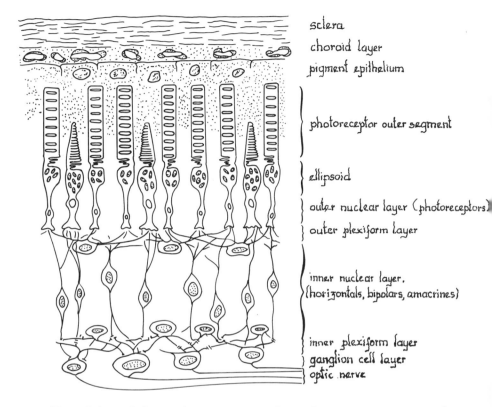

sclera

choroid layer

pigment epithelium

photoreceptor outer segment

ellipsoid

outer nuclear layer (photoreceptors)

outer plexiform layer

inner nuclear layer,
(horizontals, bipolars, amacrines)

inner plexiform layer

ganglion cell layer

optic nerve

Fig. 2.1:   Schematic representation of a transverse section through a retina. See Fig. 1.5 for a photomicrographic view.

cells.   The terms rods and cones were derived initially from the shape of the outer segments. Cells with outer segments of uniform and similar diameter as the inner segments (i.e. cylindrical) were designated rods; while cells with outer segments which tapered from the vitread to sclerad direction (i.e. conical) were called cones. Later, further anatomical and physiological features were employed in the characterisation of these cells (Table 2.1; Fig. 2.2).

The outer segments are of special interest because it is in these membranous discs that the visual pigment (that pigment which interacts with photons to initiate the visual process) is located. Generally, the rod outer segment consists of stacked discs which are isolated from the plasma membrane, although occasionally the lower discs may appear 'open' and continuous with the cell

Table 2.1: Comparison of the morphological features of rods and
cones.

ROD	CONE
Long, cylindrical outer segment with a disc repeat period of approximately 18,5-22 nm.	Tapered (conical) outer segment with a lamella repeat period of approximately 22,0-25,5 nm.
Outer segment plasma membrane-disc continuity limited to the basal portion of the outer segment.	Outer segment plasma membrane-lamella continuity frequently observed along the entire length of the outer segment.
Outer segment discs may be lobulated by incisions.	Outer segment lamellae are not lobulated.
Outer and inner segments of similar diameter.	Inner segment diameter usually larger than that of the outer segment.
Ellipsoid mitochondria generally less numerous and less dense.	Ellipsoid mitochondria more numerous and more closely packed.
Connecting-fibres usually long and slender.	Connecting-fibres usually shorter.
Nuclei generally sclerad of the outer plexiform layer.	Nuclei generally vitread of the external limiting membrane.
Synaptic pedicle usually spherical with one to several units per pedicle.	Synaptic pedicle usually conical with a broad base and 12-25 synaptic units per pedicle.

membrane. It is the discontinuity between the rod discs and plasma
membrane which resulted in the speculation that a 'transmitter' is
necessary to convey the changes in the visual pigment, evoked by
the absorption of photons, to the plasma membrane; because it is
this membrane which is hyperpolarised by light. Calcium and
cyclic nucleotides (cyclic adenosine 3',5'-monophosphate; cyclic
guanosine 3',5'-monophosphate) have been proposed as candidates

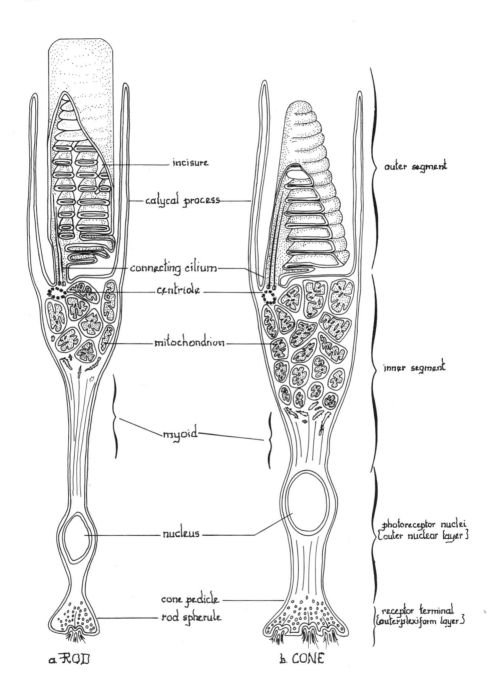

incisure

calycal process

connecting cilium

centriole

mitochondrion

myoid

nucleus

cone pedicle
rod spherule

outer segment

inner segment

photoreceptor nuclei
(outer nuclear layer)

receptor terminal
(outerplexiform layer)

a. ROD   b. CONE

for the role of transmitter (Chapter 10). Each flattened disc is hollow, and the space between the inner surfaces of the disc is about 2,5 nm under isotonic conditions. X-ray diffraction measurements have shown that the intradiscal space changes with osmotic variation (Blaurock & Wilkins, 1969). Each disc is about 15 nm thick and separated from its neighbour by the same thickness, thus making the disc-disc repeat distance 30 nm. While the disc membranes of rods appear pinched-off from the plasma membrane (closed or discontinuous) those of the cones remain continuous (open) with the plasma membrane from which they are formed (Fig. 2.2). A further morphological difference between rods and cones is the presence of incisures in the former (Fig. 2.2).

The Inner Segment

The inner segment extends from the base of the outer segment (to which it is connected by a modified cilium - the connecting cilium) to the outer limiting membrane. The apex of the inner segment gives rise to the microvillous processes. These processes have no known function.

Connecting Cilium:

The connecting cilium which connects the outer segment to the inner segment has a structure typical of cilia in the animal kingdom. Within the cilium there are at least nine tubules, usually there are eighteen arranged in pairs forming two concentric rings. The central pair of tubules is generally absent. These ciliary tubules enter the outer segment at the base of the groove formed by the disc incisions, and in the rods may run throughout the length of the groove. At the vitread end the tubules penetrate the apical portion of the inner segment and end in a centriole or basal body. A second centriole may sometimes be seen perpendicular to the first, this centriole is usually absent from the photoreceptors of some deep-sea fishes. In addition, the connecting cilium may be practically non-existent (e.g. a diurnal gecko - Pedler & Tansley, 1963; abnormal photoreceptors of man, mouse, rabbit - Tokuyasu & Yamada, 1960). The ciliary tubules are seen in the visual cell

Fig. 2.2: Diagrammatic representation of a transverse section through rod (a) and cone (b) photoreceptors showing some of the morphological differences between these cells. See Table 1 for details.

before the differentiation of the outer segment and it is thought
that they act as a site of intracellular induction for the plasma
membrane invaginations that form the outer segment discs
(Tokuyasu & Yamada, 1960).

Ellipsoid:

The distal portion of the inner segment, the ellipsoid, is
apparently the metabolic centre of the photoreceptor as it houses
an accumulation of mitochondria; cone ellipsoids generally contain
more mitochondria than rod ellipsoids.   In addition, there is an
apparent size and structure stratification among cone mitochondria
in routinely fixed retinal preparations (glutaraldehyde/osmium
tetroxide; Fig. 2.3).

The inner segments of cones of certain vertebrates (e.g.
amphibians, reptiles, birds) may contain oil droplets at their apices
(Fig. 2.4).   These droplets (generally coloured in diurnal vertebrates
and colourless in nocturnal ones) are thought to be of mitochondrial

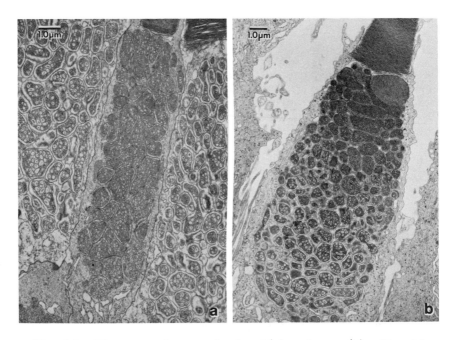

Fig. 2.3: Electron micrograph of rod (a) and cone (b) ellipsoids
of Salvelinus fontinalis illustrating the gradient of mitochondria.

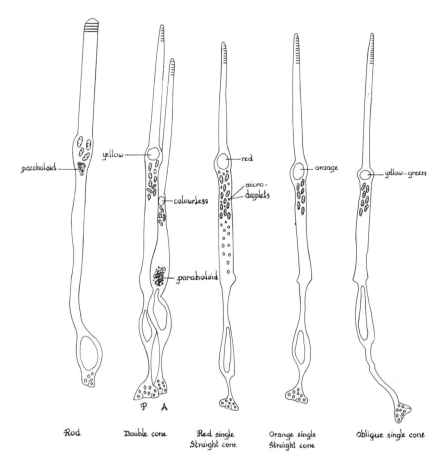

Fig. 2.4: Photoreceptors in the red region of the pigeon retina showing the location of the paraboloid; and the location and colour of oil droplets.
P   -principal member of double cone;
A   -accessory member of double cone.
(After Mariani & Leure-duPree, 1978)

origin (Berger, 1966). The role of these droplets is uncertain, but they have been suggested to act as colour filters (see Chapter 9); and as lenses by concentrating incident light onto the outer segments.

Another organelle occasionally found in the inner segments of certain fishes, amphibians, reptiles and birds is the paraboloid (Fig.

2.4). It is a spherical or oval body made up of a dense outer rim and a lighter centre. This organelle, which consists primarily of glycogen, lies between the ellipsoid and myoid. Walls (1942) suggested that the paraboloid and the ellipsoid are refractile in the living state and may affect the passage of light.

Myoid:

The bridge which connects the ellipsoid to the nucleus is termed the myoid. In certain species (e.g. lower vertebrates) this region is contractile and responsible for the radial movements of photoreceptors in response to illumination - retinomotor or photomechanical movements (Chapter 5). In species exhibiting retinomotor movements, cone myoids contract in light and elongate in darkness; while the converse holds for rod myoids. The mechanism underlying this phenomenon is unknown, but micro-tubules and microfilaments are thought to be involved.

The Outer Nuclear Layer

In duplex retinas, the nuclei of cones tend to be located adjacent to the outer limiting membrane while those of the rods occupy a more vitread position. Occasionally, the cone nuclei may lie deeper in the outer nuclear layer while the rod nuclei appear more sclerad (e.g. frog), however this arrangement is atypical.

The Receptor Terminal

The synaptic bases of the visual cells are called spherules if they are small and round; and pedicles if they are somewhat larger and present a flattened base to the second order neurones (horizontal and bipolar cells) (Fig. 2.5). Generally, the endings of rods are termed spherules and those of cones, pedicles; however all photoreceptor terminals of the pigeon and frog qualify as pedicles despite the presence of both rods and cones (see Cohen, 1972). It is nevertheless generally true that rods have smaller pedicles than cones. Numerous vesicles (30 - 50 nm in diameter) termed synaptic vesicles are present within the pedicles. These vesicles are thought to function as carriers for neurohumors. Contact between the photoreceptor and second order neurones occurs at the bases of the receptor terminal. Typically it is characterised by a non-membranous electron-dense structure on the presynaptic side - the synaptic ribbon. This structure appears anchored in a narrow extension of the receptor terminal cytoplasm - the synaptic ridge.

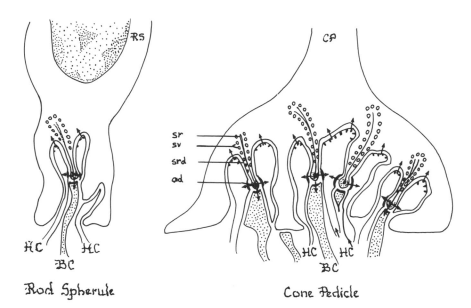

Rod Spherule   Cone Pedicle

Fig. 2.5: Schematic representation of the synaptic complexes in the vicinity of a synaptic ribbon (sr) in a cone pedicle (CP) and rod spherule (RS).
→   -direction of synaptic transmission;
HC -horizontal cell;
BC -bipolar cell;
sr   -synaptic ribbon
sv   -synaptic vesicle;
srd -synaptic ribbon ridge;
ad   -arciform density.
(After Wagner, 1978)

The distal part of the ridge shows a characteristic swelling which encloses an electron-dense, bar-like structure separated from the synaptic ribbon by a small gap - arciform density (Fig. 2.5). The ribbon synapse is contacted by processes of horizontal and bipolar cell dendrites.   Generally, horizontal cell processes flank the synaptic ridge while the bipolar cell process is located below the apex of the ridge - this configuration is termed triad (Dowling & Boycott, 1966).

General

A photoreceptor may appear single or associated with another member of its kind; when both members are identical they are called twin (or equal double) photoreceptors and when different they are called unequal double photoreceptors. This distinction was based initially on strictly morphological observations, however it was later suggested that twin photoreceptors should also possess identical visual pigments (Levine & MacNichol, 1979). Twin/double cones (general occurence) and rods (more limited distribution; e.g. nocturnal lizards) are known to occur. Cones are normally considered the older and more primitive of the two photoreceptors as cones are associated with diurnal vision and the primitive ancestors of the vertebrate stock were diurnal in habit. Rods are thought to represent the transmuted cones of these diurnal ancestors. It is also interesting to note that the retinas of most teleost embryos examined prior to metamorphosis contained only cones, rods appearing only at metamorphosis (Blaxter & Jones, 1967; Blaxter & Staines, 1970). An exception to the above is found in the eel. Larvae of Anguilla anguilla were found to contain only rod-like photoreceptors while post-metamorphic juveniles were found to display a duplex (rods and cones) retina (see Pankhurst, 1984).

In vertebrates, cones predominate in the retinas of diurnal species; and rods in nocturnal ones. Strictly diurnal (e.g. lizards, squirrels) and nocturnal (e.g. bush baby) species possess pure cone and pure rod retinas, respectively. This observation, first noted in 1866 by Schultze led to the suggestion that rods operate at low light intensities and cones at high light intensities; the latter also being responsible for colour vision. This formulation which was subsequently enlarged and modified by von Kries (1896) was based primarily on the difference in human day- and night- vision, and designated the 'Duplicity Theory'. Although there has been much criticism of the duplicity theory since its postulation it has stood the test of time and is true in a broad sense.

Further properties attributed to the different photoreceptors are sensitivity and acuity. Visual sensitivity, the ability to appreciate low light intensities, is the property of rods; while visual acuity or resolving power, the ability to distinguish fine detail is the property of cones. These functions are dealt with in a later chapter (Chapter 8).

Secondary (Intermediate) Neurones

The main members of the intermediate neuronal layer are the bipolar, horizontal and amacrine cells (Figs. 1.5, 2.1). The bipolar cells, which send processes into both synaptic layers (outer and inner plexiform layers), occupy the middle and distal third of the inner nuclear layer. The horizontal cells occupy one or more layers near the first synaptic (outer plexiform) layer; while the amacrine cells have a similar relationship with the second synaptic (inner plexiform) layer. In some instances bipolar and amacrine cell bodies may be displaced, the former to the layer of the outer nuclear layer and the latter to the inner plexiform or ganglion cell layers. In addition, glial cells of Müller (Müller cells) may also be observed among the intermediate neurones (Fig. 1.5).

Bipolar Cells

Bipolar cells make contact with photoreceptor cells sclerally and ganglion cells vitreally. They are the channels through which visual impulses must traverse on their way to ganglion cells before leaving the retina to be conveyed to the brain. Thus they have an important role in determining visual acuity.

The retinas of most vertebrates contain at least two distinct types of bipolar cells - the large bipolars and the small bipolars. The large bipolar, with a broader and deeper dendritic tree, is associated with rods; while the small bipolar is associated with cones.

Further distinction and characterisation of bipolar cells have been made. Parthe (1972) observed five types of bipolar cells (two associated with rods and three associated with cones) in Golgi preparations of several species of marine teleosts. In addition, in the fovea of the chameleon and birds there is a variety of bipolar cells which is unusually small. This bipolar cell which may contact only one cone is termed monosynaptic or midget. This type of cell has also been observed in the retinas of man, monkey and dog. Electron microscopic studies of Golgi preparations showed that there are two types of midget bipolars, as well as other bipolars including the mop, brush and flat-top varieties. In addition, Golgi-EM studies (Kolb, 1970; Kolb et al., 1969; Stell, 1967) showed the exact connexions of bipolars. They showed that the bipolars for rods send dendrites also to cones; the diffuse flat-topped bipolars are connected exclusively to cones; and the diffuse mop bipolars of primates are connected only to rods. Displaced bipolars with cell bodies in the proximal region of photoreceptor nuclei are found in birds, reptiles, amphibians and lower fishes. There is no remarkable difference between these and the other bipolars except for the displaced cell body.

Horizontal Cells

Horizontal cells contact the photoreceptors in the first synaptic layer and serve in the lateral transmission of the visual signal. They are unusually large, polygonal or stellate cells which form a distinctly continuous, but perforated layer just proximal to the first synaptic layer to which they send dendrites.

The number of rows of horizontal cells vary with the type and proportion of photoreceptors present within the retina. In retinas with an equal number of rods and cones there are generally two rows of horizontal cells. The dendrites of the first row (external or sclerad type) end at the level of the cone pedicles while those of the second row (intermediate or vitread type) end at the level of the rod spherules. The size and number of horizontal cells increase with the proportion of rods, and in retinas with a high ratio of rods there may be as many as four rows of horizontal cells.

Amacrine Cells

The amacrine cells bear a similar relationship within the second synaptic layer as horizontal cells do within the first. Amacrine cells, except for the displaced varieties, have cell bodies located within the proximal position of the intermediate neuronal layers, and they have processes extending into the second synaptic (inner plexiform) layer where they contact ganglion cells.

These cells are more diversified and numerous than horizontal cells; however, less is known about them. They are classified as stratified and diffuse or unstratified according to the nature of their processes. Stratified amacrines have the main branches of their processes ramifying in the same planar level; they are called unistratified if the ramifications are in a single level and bi- or multi-stratified when in two or more levels. On the other hand, the main branches of diffuse or unstratified amacrines end or synapse without respect to stratification within the synaptic layer.

Ganglion Cells

Ganglion cells are the final cell type through which visual impulses traverse before leaving the retina. Dendrites of these cells contact bipolars within the second synaptic layer and most likely determine the properties of the centre of the receptive fields.

Ganglion cells are classified according to the size of their dendritic fields. The updated description (Boycott & Dowling, 1969) of primate ganglion cells is as follows: midget - with a dendrite field of 10 μm or less, found in all regions of the retina; diffuse - with a dendritic field of 30-75 μm, found in all regions of the retina but which is larger in the periphery of the retina; stratified diffuse - commonly observed cell which ramifies in the second synaptic layer, most often distal and least often proximal; unistratified - with variable dendritic field, but generally around 200 μm; and displaced - with the cell bodies in the layer of the intermediate neurones, this cell type is commonly observed in birds. In addition there is another type of ganglion cell - biplexiform or interplexiform. This cell has its cell body located in the ganglion cell layer; an axon in the nerve fibre layer; dendrites in the inner plexiform layer (postsynaptic to amacrine cell processes and bipolar cell axon terminals); and also processes which extend to the outer plexiform layer (postsynaptic to rod photoreceptor terminals as the central element at the ribbon complex) Mariani, 1982). Thus this biplexiform cell represents a means whereby the commonly described interneurone circuitry of the vertebrate retina could be bypassed.

Little is known about the interconnexions between ganglion cells.

Electrophysiological Evidence of Retinal Characteristics

When the eye is stimulated by light it responds electrically by a difference in potential between the cornea and the back of the eye. This is known as the electroretinogram (ERG). The ERG is usually recorded by placing a pair of electrodes on opposite sides of the retina (excised eyes or isolated retina); however it is possible to gain recordings of the intact eye by placing one electrode on the cornea and the other on the forehead. The ERG may differ in shape according to the species and its state of adaptation as well as to the stimulus (Fig. 2.6). Typically it starts with a cornea-negative deflexion (a-wave) followed by a cornea-positive one (b-wave). At the termination of the light stimulus there occurs

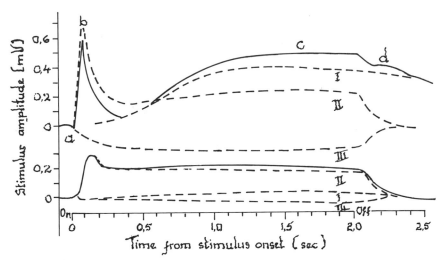

Fig. 2.6: Granit's (1933) analysis of the electroretinogram showing how it may be analysed into three processes: **PI, PII** and PIII. They add together to produce an electrogram with the **a, b** and **c** waves, and as an off-effect labelled **d. PI** is primarily responsible for the **c**-wave, **PII** for the **b**-wave, and **PIII** for the **a**- and **d**-waves. The upper graph is an analysis of the response to a bright stimulus; while the lower graph is for a dim stimulus.
(After   Armington, 1974)

another deflexion (**d**-wave), this may be cornea-negative or cornea-positive depending on the species.   In the dark-adapted retina, there is also a very slow cornea-positive deflexion (**c**-wave).

Several attempts have been made to analyse the ERG in terms of its components, but the analysis by Granit (P I, P II, P III; see Granit, 1947) is the one most generally accepted (Fig. 2.6). The introduction of the microelectrode (Tomita, 1950) enabled a more direct localisation of the ERG components by means of depth recording within the retina itself.

P I: P I of Granit (**c**-wave) is a slow cornea-positive potential which originates in the pigment epithelium layer of the retina. It is thought to manifest the metabolic interactions between the photoreceptors and pigment epithelium cells. However, as P I is not discerned in pure cone retinas it is considered to represent a process related primarily to the rod system.

P II: The fast, cornea-positive potential, P II (b-wave), reflects the activity of cells in the inner nuclear layer (bipolar, horizontal, amacrine).   Indeed a large b-wave is recorded from retinas whose inner nuclear layer is well developed.   Among the cells in this layer the bipolars are radial, with the horizontal and amacrine cells being lateral.   The bipolars are suspected to be the main contributors to P II.

Recent intracellular microelectrode studies have demonstrated three response types among cells in the inner nuclear layer: i) the ON type which represents a depolarisation with light; ii) the OFF type which represents a hyperpolarisation with light; and iii) the ON-OFF type which exhibits a phasic depolarisation at both the turning on and the turning off of the light stimulus. The first two response types originate mostly in bipolar cells and are usually dependent on the stimulus pattern; while the third response type originates in the amacrine cells and is independent of the photic stimuli and often spikes on the depolarising phases.

P III: P III is a fast, cornea-negative potential and consists of two subcomponents. The distal P III, originates in the receptors of cold-blooded animals, and is identified with the mammalian late receptor potential.   The proximal P III, on the other hand, is localised in the inner nuclear layer and is thought to be due to the hyperpolarising response of bipolar cells.

Applications

Receptors make synaptic contact with bipolar cells which then contact the ganglion cells whose axons leave the retina as the optic nerve. In the first synaptic layer, where receptors contact bipolar cells, the bipolar endings are flanked by processes of horizontal cells while the amacrines provide the lateral interconnexions at the ganglion and bipolar cell contacts in the second synaptic layer.

ERG

Although the ERG arises largely from the region of the bipolar cells the classical ERG is the sum of several different responses in the eye and as such cannot be used for detailed investigations of colour vision. As mentioned above, the components of the ERG (P I, P II, P III) respond with differential patterns of excitation and inhibition, furthermore the activities of different stages of processing are superimposed and mutually mask one another. However, with appropriate techniques some aspects of colour vision can be examined by the ERG. One of the basic problems is the elimination of rod responses which otherwise predominate. Riggs et al. (1966) were able to compute relative response functions for three independent chromatic mechanisms in man by using rapid shifts from one colour to another within a bright field of alternately coloured bars. There are however further complications, different parts of the ERG waveform apparently do not have the same spectral sensitivity; in the carp, the a-wave is largely green-sensitive while the b-wave receives inputs from red-absorbing cones; and in the goldfish, locally recorded ERG has a green-sensitive slow component and a red-sensitive oscillatory process. Nevertheless, the ERG still has the advantage that it can be measured from both human and animal subjects, but at present its complexities are sufficient to make interpretation difficult and to limit its use to experimental investigations.

Cone Potentials

Recording from single cones is technically difficult but it is still possible through the use of very fine micro-electrodes. Cones respond to light by hyperpolarisation (increase in electronegativity inside). By using lights of specific wavelengths it was found that the action spectra in a trichromatic species (e.g. goldfish) fall into three groups corresponding to the sensitivities of one of the three photopigments.

S-Potentials

S-potentials come from structures at the level of bipolar cells. This is a slow graded potential which is maintained for the duration of a light stimulus. The S-potential is found in most vertebrate eyes and does possess certain features of interest for colour vision. There are two categories of responses: the L (luminosity)-type which represents some degree of hyperpolarisation to all wavelengths; and the C (chromatic)-type which exhibits opponent spectral responses - responding with hyperpolarisation to one portion of the spectrum and depolarisation to others (Fig. 2.7). Thus the C-type response represents the first stage at which wavelength (colour) discrimination can take place, whereas the L-type response cannot by itself provide such a basis for discrimination.

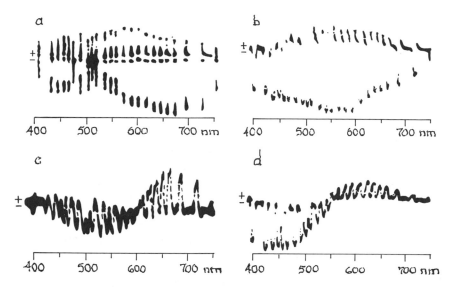

Fig. 2.7: S-potentials. Typical 'luminosity' (**L: a, b**) and 'chromaticity' (**C: c** = R-G response, **d** = B-Y response). Record **a** is taken from a retina from which the pigment layer was not removed; **b, c,** and **d** taken from another retina from which the pigment layer was removed. All responses 10 mV, but no resting potential in **a** which was presumably extracellular; **b, c** and **d** had resting potentials 20 mV (negative) and were presumably intracellular.
(From MacNichol & Svaetichin, 1958)

The anatomical sources of the S-potentials are not entirely clear. The L-type response is usually attributed to the horizontal cells. The location of the C-type response is however less well defined. This response was originally ascribed to the amacrine cells, but the method of dye-injection, following recordings, by Kaneko (1970) showed that C-type responses also originate from horizontal cells.

Ganglion Cells

Responses transmitted from the retina along the optic nerve are spike potentials. Ganglion cells, in several vertebrate retinas, generally maintain some firing rate even in the absence of specific stimulation. Thus responses of ganglion cells to specific stimulation can be either increase (excitation) or decrease (inhibition) of the spontaneous rate. Traditionally these have been referred to as the ON and OFF responses.

In species with well developed colour vision there are two categories of ganglion cell responses which are analogous to those of the S-potential. There are the spectrally non-opponent cells which respond with either excitation or inhibition to all wavelengths - ascribed as pure ON and OFF cells; as well as spectrally opponent cells whose responses depend on the wavelength of the stimulus. The non-opponent cells constitute about one-third of the cells and they are divided equally between cells responding to all parts of the spectrum with excitation and inhibition. Spectrally opponent cells may be divided into four types on the basis of their response to specific wavelengths: +R-G (red excitation and green inhibition) and its converse (+G-R); and +Y-B (yellow excitation and blue inhibition) and its converse (+B-Y). These names describe the spectral loci of peak excitation and inhibition without necessarily saying how inputs from the various cones were combined to give the response types. There is no marked difference in the relative numbers of the four types of cells although +G-R and +R-G are most numerous with +B-Y being the least common. The two types of responses (spectrally opponent and non-opponent) have been recorded from the retinal ganglion cells of several vertebrates including the goldfish, carp, macaque monkey and the ground squirrel; species possessing well-developed colour vision. In species with less well-developed colour vision, similar responses have been observed, however the spectrally opponent cells are less prevalent and less diversified.

Purkinje Shift

The Purkinje shift or Purkinje phenomenon is the change in spectral sensitivity which occurs when a light-adapted eye is allowed to dark-adapt or vice versa. It was first described by the Czech physiologist in 1825. The light-adapted human eye was found to be most sensitive to the yellow region of the spectrum while the dark-adapted eye was most sensitive to blue-green. It was later established that the maximum absorption of rhodopsin (rod pigment) corresponded to the human dark-adapted visibility of approximately 500 nm (König, 1894) and that the sensitivity of the light-adapted eye was greatest around 550 nm, the maximum luminosity of the visual spectrum (Gibson & Tyndall, 1923-24; Kohlrausch, 1931). This shift in spectral sensitivity, when an animal moves from dark surroundings to a brighter one or vice versa, has no bearing on colour vision, instead it illustrates the involvement of two types of photoreceptors (rods and cones) in scotopic and photopic vision. Thus, the Purkinje shift is not found in pure cone (e.g. squirrel) or pure rod (e.g. nocturnal gecko) retinas, neither is it present in foveal vision. It is, however, present in the mixed retinas of the cat, frog, tench, carp, pigeon, starling and chicken (Fig. 2.8).

The Purkinje shift can be demonstrated either by behavioural or electrophysiological means in animals whose retinas contain a fair proportion of rods and cones. In the latter method, recordings from bipolar and ganglion cells can be used to demonstrate this shift. The b-wave of the ERG as a function of wavelength in an equal energy spectrum showed that the maximal b-waves occurred at 507 nm for the dark-adapted retina and 560 nm for the light-adapted one (Armington, 1955; Granit & Munsterhjelm, 1937;

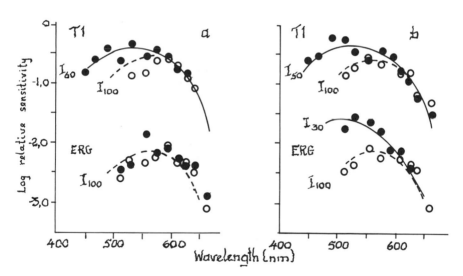

Fig. 2.8: Relative spectral sensitivity for two chickens. The figure compares the sensitivity of responses obtained at the retina (ERG) and at the optic tectum (TI) of the chicken. Note that one chicken showed no Purkinje shift at the retina, yet displayed one at the tectum (a). The other showed a larger shift at the retina than at the tectum (b).
● -dark-adapted eye;
o -light-adapted eye.
(From Armington & Crampton, 1958)

Granit & Wrede, 1937). The action potentials from ganglion cells showed that as the retina dark-adapted the maximal nerve impulse discharge was shifted to shorter wavelengths (504 nm for toad) and to longer wavelengths (558 nm for toad) as the retina light-adapted (Lipetz, 1962).

Movement Perception

The perception of movement is one of the most vital and fundamental functions of the eye. Species which feed on live animals can starve to death while surrounded by dead prey. Frogs and toads will feed on food (natural and non-natural) that is moving, or is in an environment which is moving. Perch will only snap at moving bait; here the direction of movement is the determining factor although if the movement is too rapid they will not respond. Microelectrode recordings from ganglion cells of the retinas of the rabbit, frog and pigeon have shown that certain ganglion cells respond to movement in one direction only.

The speed of movement is important because if the movement is too rapid the image resting on the retina will not be long enough to register a visual sensation; while if it is too slow the actual movement is not perceived. Thus, the perception of movement is dependent on the fineness of the retinal "grain", movement being perceived only if the image moves from one receptive field of the optic nerve fibre to another - the smaller the receptive field the lower is the threshold of movement which can be appreciated. This would mean that perception of movement is more acute in a cone retina than in a rod retina as the receptive field is smaller in the former. In general, the higher the visual acuity the more acute the perception of movement.

Tied in to the perception of movement is the phenomenon of the persistence of vision. A transient retinal stimulus does not cease to exist immediately after the stimulus is removed, instead it persists for a short interval depending on the state of adaptation of the eye and the intensity of the stimulus. If a black and white sectored disc is rotated the individual sectors can be recognised if the rotation is slow enough; as the speed of rotation is increased the disc will appear to flicker due to the mergence of the persisting image of one sector with that of the next. If the speed of rotation is further increased the perception of movement will be lost and the disc will appear as uniformly grey. The speed of rotation of the disc at which the flickering just disappears is known as the flicker fusion frequency (FFF) and it is a good indication of the ability of the eye to follow movement. FFF is higher for cones than for rods as cone reactions are faster. In conjunction with this, FFF is not only higher in light-adapted retinas but it also increases with increasing light intensities (Fig. 2.9). This once again illustrates that cones perceive movement better than rods and that light-adaptation is an advantage.

FFF can be measured by training the subject to react to a rotating disc while ignoring a stationary one. Thus the speed of rotation of a black and white sectored disc which does not evoke a response in the test subject is the FFF of that animal. Another method is to use the optomotor reaction. Here the animal is placed in a hollow rotating cylinder painted with black and white vertical stripes. The animal will react (e.g. turn its eyes, head or whole body) in the direction of the movement in order to maintain the image stationary on its retina.   When the speed of rotation matches the FFF of the test subject it will cease to react because the cylinder will now appear stationary. These methods of determining FFF have also been employed in the study of colour vision by painting the sectors/stripes in two different colours.

A third method employed in FFF measurement is the ERG. In the presence of a slow flicker the retina responds to each stimulus with distinct waves (a-, b-, c- and d-waves), however as the flicker rate is increased the waves get closer and closer together until

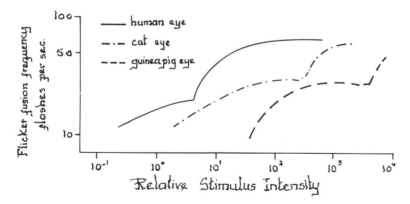

Fig. 2.9: A plot of electroretinal flicker fusion frequency as a function of stimulus intensity in three species. The data for all three subjects show a discontinuity that marks the transition from scotopic to photopic function.
(From Dodt, 1954)

they finally fuse together to produce a prolonged positive potential, this corresponds to the FFF of the species under observation (Fig. 2.10). This property of the retina may also be employed in the measurement of colour vision. This may be achieved by substituting the light stimulus with a light of a specific wavelength and measuring its flickering effect on the waves of the ERG.

In general, the faster the movement of an animal the better its perception of movement needs to be. At moderate intensities the FFF for the human fovea of a light-adapted retina is 50 cycles per second while that of the peripheral retina is 20 cycles per second. This once again illustrates the difference in the speed of response of rods and cones. The pure rod retina of the guinea-pig

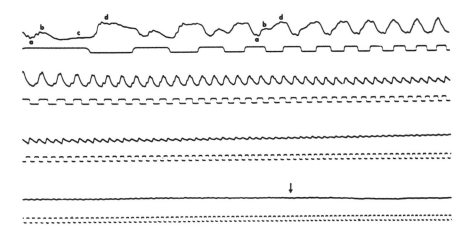

Fig. 2.10: The response of the salmon retinogram to an intermittent light stimulus of increasing frequency. At low frequencies of stimulation the individual waves as well as the ripples are distinguishable - polyphasic (a-, b-, c- and d-waves). As the frequency increases the a-wave becomes larger and the distance between the b- and d-waves decreases until the two appear as a single peak - diphasic. As the frequency is further increased the diphasic ERG changes in shape to a straight line. Intensity of the stimulating light and temperature influence the flicker ERG - both high light intensities and temperature increase the flicker fusion. The above flicker fusion of the salmon (Arrow) was 96 cycles. sec^{-1} at 25°C and with a 390 ft-c stimulating source.
(After Hanyu & Ali, 1964)

shows a maximum FFF of 45 - 50 cycles per second at maximum light intensity, while for the pure cone retina of the ground squirrel the figure is over 100 cycles per second.

3

VISUAL PIGMENTS

Light is able to stimulate directly the radial net of the sea urchin; but in vertebrates light has no effect on the optic nerve. In order to trigger the discharges in the optic nerve there must be a light-sensitive mediating mechanism. In the vertebrate eye this is achieved by the photostimulation of the visual pigments. Rhodopsin when photostimulated undergoes a series of spontaneous reactions which ultimately results in stable products. These sequences of events do not require enzymatic or metabolic energy. On the other hand, the regeneration of the visual pigment from the product of reaction is energy consuming. The photoactivation and regeneration of the visual pigment, termed the visual cycle (Wald, 1935) is illustrated in Fig. 3.1.

In rods, these pigments are located on the disc membranes of the outer segments which are isolated from the plasma membrane; while in cones, where the outer segments are transverse infoldings of the plasma membrane, the visual pigments are part of the continuous membrane which separates the intracellular from the extracellular space (Fig. 3.2). These pigments appear to move about freely on the surface of the bilayer membrane, exhibiting both rotational and translational motions. The distribution of the visual pigment mass within the membrane bilayer is a matter of controversy. Most studies have been conducted using rod outer segments. X-ray studies of these membranes indicate that much of the pigment lies outside the membrane while part is anchored in the outer-half of the bilayer (Fig. 3.2). Freeze-fracture analyses, on the other hand, indicate that rhodopsin may span the entire thickness of the disc membrane (Fig. 3.2). This trans-membrane nature of rhodopsin has been demonstrated by iodination studies on disc membranes and reconstituted vesicles (Fung & Hubbell, 1978).

43

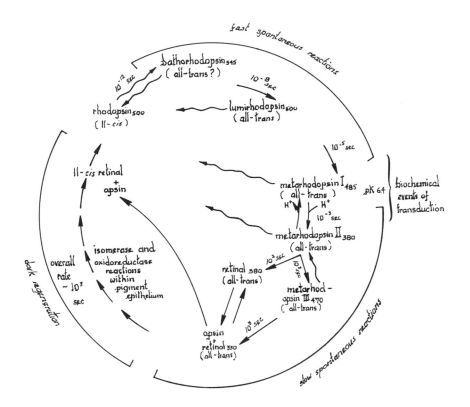

Fig. 3.1: The visual cycle of rat rhodopsin. Photochemical reactions are represented by wavy lines; dark reactions (spontaneous or enzymatic) by straight lines. The λ_{max} of each intermediate appears as a subscript, with the conformation of its chromophore in parentheses. Note, the decay of metarhodopsin II can form either metarhodopsin III or "retinal", the latter being a chromophore-protein complex that is spectrally indistinguishable from free retinal. Both these molecules lead to formation of opsin and all-trans retinol. The latter molecule, which moves freely between the receptor cell and the pigment epithelium, is oxidised and isomerised by energy consuming dark reactions to yield 11-cis retinal. It then spontaneously reacts with opsin, which did not move beyond the confines of its membrane, to regenerate rhodopsin. The cited rate constant for the formation of each spectral intermediate refers to physiological temperatures. The rate for the rhodopsin → bathorhodopsin transition was obtained for rhodopsin solutions, and the rates for the remainder of the bleaching cycle were obtained on excised rat retinas. The

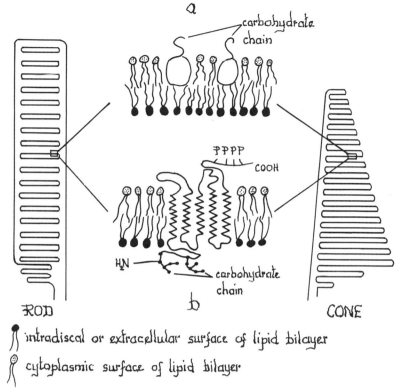

a

carbohydrate chain

PPPP

COOH

HN

carbohydrate chain

b

ROD

CONE

intradiscal or extracellular surface of lipid bilayer

cytoplasmic surface of lipid bilayer

Fig. 3.2: Proposals for the localisation of visual pigments on photoreceptor outer segments.

a - The visual pigment may lie on one side of the membrane bilayer with part of the pigment on the outside and the other part anchored within the bilayer (Hubbell, 1975).

b - The visual pigment may span the entire thickness of the membrane bilayer (Hargrave et al., 1980).

Note: In the two models (a, b) the carbohydrate chains have been placed on different surfaces of the membrane bilayer.

---

identity of the individual reactions by which all-trans retinol is converted to 11-cis retinal has been omitted. The above cycle refers to the intact eye. For an isolated retina, devoid of its pigment epithelium, dark regeneration is absent. In addition, if rhodopsin is solubilised, the kinetics of the spontaneous reactions are also altered.

(After Fein & Szuts, 1982)

The cytoplasmic (external) disc membrane surface of rhodopsin is thought to contain the carboxyl-terminal of rhodopsin, while its amino-terminal (which contains sites of carbohydrate attachment) is located at the intradiscal membrane surface (see Mas et al., 1980).

The lipid composition of vertebrate visual pigment is predominantly phospholipids which contain a high degree of unsaturated fatty acid chains. This unsaturation renders fluidity to the membrane. Although the lipid is apparently not involved in a direct linkage to the chromophore it is essential to the formation of the native visual pigment and the maintenance of its native configuration. It has been shown (Shichi, 1971; Zorn & Futterman, 1971) that incubation of 11-cis retinal with bovine opsin will not result in pigment formation unless phospholipids are present.

Biochemistry

All visual pigments are chromolipoproteins whose chromophores are thought to be derived from only two polyene aldehyde sources - 11-cis retinal (Vitamin A_1) and its 3-dehydroderivative (Vitamin A_2) (Fig. 3.3). These aldehydes are linked to protein moieties, generically called opsin, by a protonated Schiff base linkage with the **N** of an amino acid residue (ε -**N** of lysine for rhodopsin) to form visual pigments. Unlike the chromophores, the structure of opsin is unknown. However, this apoprotein is an intrinsic membrane protein with a single polypeptide chain to which two short oligosaccharide segments are attached. The names of the visual pigments are derived from the types of retinal (Vitamin A) they contain. Thus, retinal A_1 (11-cis retinal) when combined with rod opsin yields rhodopsin and when combined with cone opsin gives iodopsin. Similarly, retinal A_2 (11-cis-3-dehydroretinal) combines with rod opsin to yield porphyropsin and with cone opsin to yield cyanopsin (Fig. 3.3). The opsin alone does not absorb visible light, however, when it is combined to the chromophore (retinal), it imparts colour to the visual pigment thus formed. The fact that pigments of different species exhibit different absorption spectra is attributed to variations in the protein moiety (opsin) and hence to its interactions with the chromophore. A number of theoretical studies on the spectrum of retinal in the unprotonated and protonated forms show that protonation results in a shift to longer wavelengths. However, protonation per se is unlikely to shift the absorption significantly beyond that observed for the protonated Schiff base in solution. Thus, additional contributions are required

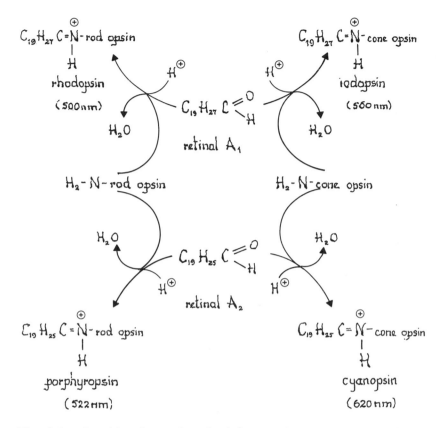

$$\overset{\oplus}{C_{19}H_{27}\,C=N-\text{rod opsin}}$$
$$|$$
$$H$$

rhodopsin

(500nm)

$$C_{19}H_{27}\,C \overset{O}{\underset{\searrow H}{=}}$$

retinal A_1

$$\overset{\oplus}{C_{19}H_{27}\,C=N-\text{cone opsin}}$$
$$|$$
$$H$$

iodopsin

(560 nm)

H_2O $H^{\oplus}$ $H^{\oplus}$ H_2O

$H_2-N-\text{rod opsin}$ $H_2-N-\text{cone opsin}$

H_2O H_2O

$$C_{19}H_{25}\,C \overset{O}{\underset{\searrow H}{=}}$$

retinal A_2

$H^{\oplus}$ $H^{\oplus}$

$$\overset{\oplus}{C_{19}H_{25}\,C=N-\text{rod opsin}}$$
$$|$$
$$H$$

porphyropsin

(522nm)

$$\overset{\oplus}{C_{19}H_{25}\,C=N-\text{cone opsin}}$$
$$|$$
$$H$$

cyanopsin

(620 nm)

Fig. 3.3: Combinations of retinal A_1 and A_2 with rod and cone opsins to yield rhodopsin, porphyropsin, iodopsin and cyanopsin.

to obtain the spectral shift observed in rhodopsin and its analogues. These are thought to come from the molecular charge distribution of the ground and excited states of the protonated Schiff base of retinal. Either positive (e.g. $-NH_3^+$) or negative (e.g. $-COO^-$) groups can produce shifts to longer or shorter wavelengths depending on their position relative to the chain (e.g. a positive charge near the carbon atom which is more negative in the ground than in the excited state would stabilise it and result in a shift to a shorter wavelength). Shifts in wavelengths may also be achieved through twisting of the chromophore. The polyene chain of retinal is quite flexible, and twists about the double bonds can be induced by the protein moiety, thus, yielding shifts to longer wavelengths. The three characteristic peaks of the absorption spectrum of rhodopsin (α, β, γ) are shown in Fig. 3.4. Of these, the γ-peak is due to protein absorption and the α- and β-peaks represent electronic transition movements. The α-peak results from a transition movement that induces electronic oscillations along the entire length of the conjugated bond, while the β-peak represents transition movements that only induce partial oscillations along the bent polyene chain.

Visual pigments may be characterised not only by the opsins and retinals they contain but also by their colour. All visual pigments are coloured, that is they do not absorb wavelengths of light equally. Spectra of visual pigments are broad and structureless and are characterised by their wavelength of maximum absorption, λ_{max}. Visual pigments which absorb green wavelengths from the middle of the spectrum appear red; while those which absorb from the blue region of the spectrum appear yellow. The λ_{max} of visual pigments from different species range from about 430 nm to 562 nm for the retinal A_1 chromophore and from 510 to 620 nm for the retinal A_2 chromophore. A further interesting point is that the plot of the number of species for a given λ_{max} vs. λ gives a curve which shows that the absorption maxima tend to cluster at discrete intervals (Dartnall & Lythgoe, 1965) (Fig. 3.5). More recently, an ultraviolet visual pigment was found to be present in the small single cones of a cyprinid fish (Japanese dace, Tribolodon hakonensis Günther) (Harosi & Hashimoto, 1983).

Methods of Study

Knowledge of the visual pigment is still scanty. The major problem is the interpretation of the large spectral shifts that occur on pigment formation and the considerable variation in the maxima of pigments differing only in the nature of the protein (opsin) to which the same chromophore (retinal) is bound. Furthermore, for any given pigment the intermediates which appear in the visual cycle have a wide range of spectral maxima (Fig. 3.1).

The spectral characteristics of visual pigments may be studied through extraction and reflexion techniques or by micro-spectrophotometry.

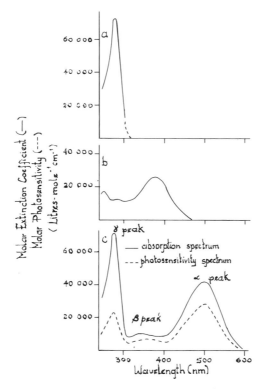

Fig. 3.4: Absorption spectra of rod opsin (a), free retinal (b), and their reaction product, rhodopsin (c).

a - The opsin spectrum was based on the γ peak of rhodopsin. Its absorption beyond 300 nm was made to fit the absorption profile of the absorbing cyclic amino acid because opsin preparations usually contain irremovable chromophore contaminants that strongly absorb in this part of the spectrum.

b - Absorption spectrum of 11-cis retinal in ethanol.

c - Absorption spectrum (———) and photosensitivity spectrum (- - -) of cattle rhodopsin solubilised with the detergent ammonyx-LO.

(After Ebrey & Honig, 1975)

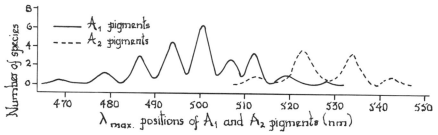

Fig. 3.5: The relationship between the spectral distribution of A_1 and A_2 pigments in teleost fishes. The data for A_1 pigments are derived from those fishes which only possess A_1 pigments; the data for A_2 pigments are not restricted, they include all fishes that possess A_2 pigments, some of which have A_1 pigments as well.
(After Dartnall & Lythgoe, 1965)

Extraction Technique

Visual pigments are membrane proteins with hydrophobic regions, thus detergents (solubilisers) are required to bring the pigments into solutions. Detergents are amphipathic molecules, i.e. they contain both polar (hydrophilic) and non-polar (hydrophobic) regions, which when in solution form micelles. The interior of the micelle contains the hydrophobic region of the molecule. Detergents extract rhodopsin from photoreceptor membranes by incorporating membrane fragments into the micelles. Not all detergents are equally effective in extracting rhodopsin, especially if undenatured pigments are required. Kühne, in 1878, showed that this may be achieved through the use of the natural anionic detergent - bile salts (mixture of sodium glycholate and taurocholate). Later, digitonin and Triton X-100 were introduced by Tansley (1931) and Crescitelli (1967), respectively, for this purpose. Still more recently, a synthetic detergent derived from cholic acid, 3-((3-cholamidopropyl) dimethylammonio)-1-propane-sulfonate (CHAPS), has been introduced for the study of visual pigments (Kropf, 1982). An ideal detergent should not alter:- (i) the absorption spectrum of rhodopsin; (ii) the rate of formation of rhodopsin when opsin and 11-cis retinal are mixed; (iii) the thermal stability of rhodopsin, a temperature of 60° C must be exceeded before temperature affects rhodopsin attached to disc membrane (Hubbard, 1958).

The visual pigments are highly photolabile and consequently the extraction procedures must be carried out under conditions necessary for developing photographic films (illuminated by dim red light) or infrared illumination. The eyes are dissected from animals dark-adapted for at least 12 hours prior to the experiment and the cornea and lens removed. This ensures that the concentration of visual pigment in the retina is at its maximum as well as ease of separation of the retina from the pigment epithelium in species which exhibit photomechanical movements. Care should be taken to handle the retina gently at all times. The retina is then isolated, and blood washed away gently with the buffer solution. Whole retinas or isolated photoreceptor outer segments may be employed for pigment extraction.

Whole Retinas

Isolated retinas are pooled and ground together in phosphate buffer (1/15 M; pH 6,3 - 7) and centrifuged at 30 000g. The supernatant is discarded and the residue ground with a small volume of detergent solution. Next the mixture is left to extract for 2 - 3 hours at $4°$ C, after which it is centrifuged. The supernatant (visual pigment extract) is then pipetted off and assayed. The residue is re-extracted with detergent, centrifuged and the supernatant assayed as before. These steps are repeated until all the rhodopsin has been extracted. Extracts may also be pooled and assayed together, however, successive extracts usually decrease in purity and it is generally best to assay the extracts individually.

Photoreceptor Outer Segments

The degree of force required to break off outer segments varies with the species. Frog photoreceptors come away very easily and it is only necessary to shake for 15 min, by hand, the retina in a tube containing a little buffer. Bovine retinas, being bulkier, must be shaken more vigorously. More violent methods have been advocated by other workers (see Davson, 1977). Alternatively, proteolytic enzymes may be employed to disintegrate the retina. The receptor suspension is spun down and washed with buffer one or more times, the supernatant is discarded while the outer segment residue is processed further.

Method I - Sucrose Flotation (a)

The residue is then taken up in a solution of sucrose (40%) at a concentration of 35 ml per 50 retinas. This suspension is then layered under neutral phosphate buffer (1/15 M) and centrifuged (30 000g, 15 - 20 min). The photoreceptor outer segments and their fragments aggregate at the interface of the sucrose and buffer solutions; and may be pipetted out, taking as little of the sucrose solution as possible. The buffer and sucrose solutions are then discarded. The outer segment suspension is diluted with about two volumes of buffer and centrifuged to sediment the outer segments. The outer segments are then made into a paste with 10 ml sucrose, layered under buffer, and centrifuged. The outer segments, at the interface, are then collected, diluted with buffer and sedimented as before. The second flotation enhances the purity and tends to remove red cell ghosts. Next, the outer segments are washed two to three times with 10 ml portions of distilled water, soaked for 10 min in alum (4% aluminium potassium sulphate in distilled water) and rewashed three times with water and once with phosphate buffer. Care should be taken to remove all traces of alum prior to the addition of the buffer as phosphate and alum reacts to yield sulphuric acid which denatures rhodopsin. The outer segments are then lyophilised and washed twice with petroleum ether (b.p. 20° - 40°) and dried gently under suction or more slowly at room temperature. This is essential in preventing flotation during subsequent extraction of rhodopsin.

Rhodopsin is finally extracted by stirring the dried, lyophilised outer segments with a detergent solution and allowing it to stand (2 - 3 hours, 4° C). After standing, the suspension is centrifuged (20 min, 30 000g) and the supernatant withdrawn. The extraction procedure is repeated to extract all the rhodopsin (usually four extractions). As with whole retinas, it is best to analyse the extracts separately because successive extracts usually lead to decreased purity.

Method II - Sucrose Flotation (b)

The outer segment residue is taken up in a 40% sucrose solution, and left in contact with the solution for 45 - 60 min in order to saturate the tissue with sucrose (final concentration will be approximately 23% sucrose). The suspension is then sedimented at 30 000g for 20 min, and the supernatant discarded. Next the sediment is homogenised thoroughly, on ice, with 40% sucrose solution (final sucrose concentration approximately 36%). The suspension is then layered under buffer and centrifuged (30 000g). The outer segments appear tightly packed at the interface of the two solutions (buffer and sucrose). The outer segment suspension is then pipetted out, resuspended in sucrose, and the flotation repeated. After the second flotation the interface (containing the outer segments) is withdrawn, washed with buffer, followed with three successive portions of distilled water, soaked in alum, and treated as in Method I.

Method III - Gradient Centrifugation

Since it is difficult to match the density of a particular outer segment to a sucrose solution, a better separation can be achieved by the centrifugation of the receptors on a sucrose density gradient. Several workers favour the use of a sucrose step-gradient (e.g. densities of 1,10; 1,11; 1,13 and 1,15 g per ml) although a linear gradient can also be made from mixtures of 25% and 45% sucrose using a two-chambered mixing device to form a density gradient from 1,09 to 1,17 g per ml.

A suspension of outer segments in dilute 25% sucrose solution is layered over the gradient and centrifuged at 65 000g for 90 min. The bands can be properly located in white light, however, the minimum possible intensity should be used and the bands withdrawn as quickly as possible. The bright red band (near the top of the tube) contains the majority of nearly pure outer segments. This band is pipetted out and treated as in Method I (i.e. washed two or three times with distilled water, soaked 10 min in alum and rewashed three times with water and once with phosphate buffer, etc.).

General

Receptor preparations or pigment extracts are subject to bacterial action, but can be kept for long periods at -30° C. In addition, there is also the problem of chemical denaturation by detergents; this is minimal for mammalian rhodopsins in digitonin, but becomes significant with other detergents, and with porphyropsins or cone pigments. Although there is little quantitative data on the stability of pigments, it is probable that the pigment is more stable when attached to the receptor than it is following extraction. Thus, if long-term storage is contemplated, it is probably better to freeze the complete retina or the receptor preparation, and to prepare the extract when required.

The extracted pigment is then introduced into an optical cell bounded by parallel faces and the absorption properties of the solution determined by reading the percentage absorption at various wavelengths. A plot of the percentage absorption versus wavelength gives the absorption spectrum of the pigment solution. This, however, suffers a drawback in that the curve is a function of concentration - the more concentrated the solution the broader will be the absorption band (Fig. 3.6a). This may be resolved by

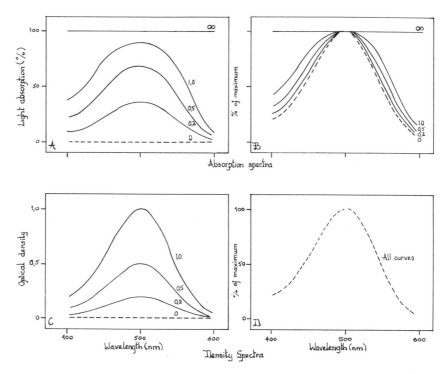

Fig. 3.6: Absorption spectra (**a, b**) and density spectra (**c, d**) of various solutions of visual purple. **b** and **d** are similar to **a** and **c**, respectively, but plotted as percentages of their maxima. (After Dartnall, 1957)

expressing the absorbance as percentage of the maximum (Fig. 3.6b); or even better as percentage of maximum optical density versus wavelength (which gives the density spectra; Fig. 3.6c, d). The latter has the advantage in that the curve of optical density when expressed as a percentage of maximum density is identical regardless of concentration (Fig. 3.6d). If coloured impurities are present in the pigment extract the difference spectrum can be obtained, this eliminates the impurities which are not affected by light. This is done by measuring the spectrum of the original extract (sample); the solution is then bleached and the spectrum once again determined (impurities). The difference in measurement of the two spectra (on a percentage basis) gives the difference spectrum. If more than one visual pigment is present in the extract their spectra may be separated by the method of partial bleaching. The pigment extract is first subjected to monochromatic light of long wavelength which bleaches the preponderant rhodopsin. The spectrum of the unaffected "residue" is then obtained prior to being subjected to bleaching lights of shorter wavelengths so as to obtain the difference spectra of the pigments present.

Pigment yields for some representable species are given in Table 2. The quantity of pigment is expressed in nanomoles (10^{-9} moles) since this can readily be related to the absorbance of the solution. The nomogram used for the calculation of the concentration of extracts of rhodopsins is given in Fig. 3.7.

Absorption properties of visual pigments prior to extraction from the visual cells may be determined by the opal-glass method

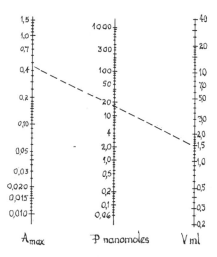

Fig. 3.7:   A nomogram giving the rhodopsin content in namomoles 10^{-9} moles of **V** ml of an extract of maximum absorbance **A**.   The left-hand scale corresponds to the absorbance of the extract and the right-hand scale the volume of the extract. The line joining a point on the left-hand scale to one on the right-hand scale cuts the centre scale at the point which gives the amount of pigment in the sample. For example, the dotted line shows that 1,5 ml of an extract of A_{max} = 0,450 contains 16,6 nmoles of rhodopsin. This is based on the assumption that λ_{max} = 40 600 $M^{-1}cm^{-1}$, which is probably applicable to most rhodopsins.
(After Knowles & Dartnall, 1977)

Table 3.1: Visual Pigment Yields From Various Species

Presumed Source	Pigment λ_{max} (nm)	Type	Yield* (nm/eye)
Man (Homo sapiens) rods	497	R	3,5
Elephant seal rods	485,5	R	23,6
(Mirounga leonina)			
Weddell seal rods	495,5	R	23,1
(Leptonychotes weddelli)			
Fur seal rods	496	R	24,8
(Arctocephalus gazella)			
Ox rods	499	R	9,9
(Bos taurus) enriched rods	499	R	16,8
Timor deer rods	498	R	7,0
(Cervus timorensis)			
Giant panda rods	494	R	1,4
(Ailuropoda melanoleuca)			
Grey squirrel rods	502	R	0,27
(Sciurus carolinensis leucotis)			
Rat rods	498	R	1,23
Rabbit rods	502	R	1,9
Crab-eating frog red rods	502	R	2,55
(Rana cancrivora) green rods	433	R	0,22
Clawed toad rods	502	R	0,09
(Xenopus laevis)	523	P	1,42
Pike (Esox lucius) (0,55 m) rods	533	P	19,4
Carp (Cyprinus carpio) rods	523	P	2,21
African lung fish rods	525	P	0,18
(Protopterus aethiopicus)			
Patterned dog fish rods	479	R	10,2
(Galeus melastomus)			
Aristostomias xenostoma unknown	553	R	1,3
	516	R	0,9

R - rhodopsin;   P - porphyropsin
* - yield calculated from the following formulae:-
   $D \times 24,6 . n^{-1}$ for A_1 pigments
   $D \times 33,3 . n^{-1}$ for A_2 pigments
   where D = absorbance of extract or combination of ex-
               tracts after adjustment to a volume of one ml
               and an optical path length of 10mm.
        n = number of eyes examined.
(After Knowles & Dartnall, 1977)

which gives results comparable to that obtained for extracted pigments (see Dartnall, 1961). In the ideal situation, a completely transparent solution, all of the light transmitted falls on the detector, **D** (Fig. 3.8:1). In a turbid solution, some of the light is transmitted forwards and still falls on the detector, while some is lost due to scattering (Fig. 3.8:2). When an opal-glass screen is placed between the cell (containing a transparent solution) and the detector only a certain fraction of the transmitted light falls on the detector (Fig. 3.8:3). When a light scattering sample is placed in the cell, all the forward-scattered light is caught by the opal-glass screen and a constant fraction of each ray enters the detector (Fig. 3.8:4). Thus, a non-scattering reference can be used, because approximately the same amount of light enters the detector whether or not the sample in the cell is light scattering. Results of the absorbance spectra of rhodopsin, in a highly scattering suspension of frog photoreceptor cells, obtained by the opal-glass technique is shown in Fig. 3.9.

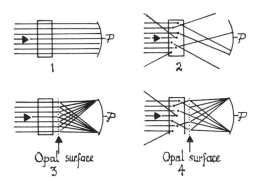

Fig. 3.8: The opal-glass method for measuring turbid solutions. A parallel beam of light passes through a sample, represented by the rectangle.

1 - When the sample is optically clear, all the light reaches the detector (P);
2 - A light-scattering sample reduces the amount of light reaching the detector;
3 - When a scattering opal glass screen is placed between the cell and the detector, the light entering the latter is again reduced;
4 - The relative reduction when a scattering sample is introduced is now very much less, the amount of light reaching the detector being nearly the same as in **3**.

(After Dartnall, 1961)

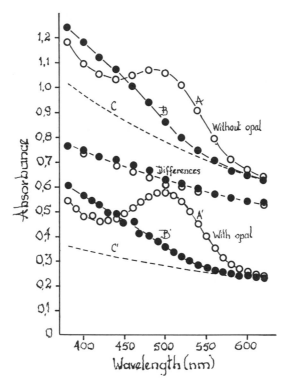

Fig. 3.9: Illustration of the opal-glass method.

Curve A: Apparent absorbance spectrum of a sucrose suspension of frog rod outer segments measured in the normal way;

Curve B: After bleaching;

Curve A': Absorbance spectrum of the same suspension measured with an opal glass screen between the cell and the detector;

Curve B': After bleaching;

Difference Curve: A - A'; B - B'. Both sets of points are displaced upwards by 0,13 for clarity.

Curves C and C': The 'difference' curve scaled up to fit curves B and B' at 620 nm. The true absorbance of the pigment is given by A - C or A' - C'.

(After Dartnall, 1961)

However, photoproducts formed when the visual pigments are bleached in situ are significantly different from those ordinarily formed in solution. Nevertheless, there is good correlation between the scotopic spectral-sensitivity curve of an animal and the density of the visual pigment extracted from rods. The matter is different when cone pigments are considered. To date, the extraction procedure when applied to cone pigments have met with limited success, only one paper (Munz & McFarland, 1975) presented presumptive photopic pigment data based on extracts.

Standard Shapes for Pigment Absorbance Spectra: The Nomograms

The Rhodopsin Nomogram

Dartnall (1953) noted that if the difference spectra is plotted on a frequency basis rather than the wavelength scale, the shapes of pigments of differing λ_{max} were almost identical. Frequency (ν) is related to wavelength by the expression:

$$\nu = c. \lambda^{-1}$$

where
λ λ is in nm
ν is in Hertz or cycles s^{-1}
c is the velocity of light ($2\ 998 \times 10^{17}\ nm.s^{-1}$)

In visual pigment studies frequency is generally expressed in wavenumbers ($\bar{\nu}\ cm^{-1}$) where

$$\bar{\nu} = \lambda^{-1}$$

Thus, green light of $\lambda = 500$ nm has a frequency of 6×10^{14} Hertz or $20\ 000\ cm^{-1}$.

The standard spectrum for rhodopsin plotted on a wave number scale (the values expressed relative to the pigment λ_{max}) is shown in Fig. 3.10. Thus for a pigment of maximum absorbance A_{max} at λ_{max}, the relative absorbance at λ_x (A_x/A_{max}), will be found corresponding to a point on the frequency scale of:-

$$\Delta\bar{\nu} = \lambda_{max}^{-1} - \lambda_x^{-1}$$

The concept of a common spectral shape was originally based on a very small number of pigments, however, it has since proved applicable to nearly all rhodopsins. A more convenient way of using the data is in the form of a nomogram that directly relates

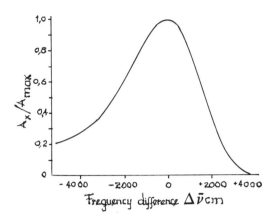

Fig. 3.10: Standard spectrum for rhodopsin pigments plotted on a wave number scale, relative to λ_{max}.
(From Wyszecki & Stiles, 1967)

A_x/A_{max} with λ_x. The rhodopsin nomogram based on the spectrum of Fig. 3.10 is shown in Fig. 3.11. The nomogram can be used in two ways.

i.   Calculation of the absorbance spectrum of a rhodopsin of given λ_{max} :- place one end of a ruler on the right-hand scale at the required λ_{max}; then rotate it about this point, the left-hand scale gives the relative absorbance corresponding to λ_x on the centre scale. For example, the upper line shows that the absorbance of a pigment of λ_{max} = 533 nm is 59% of the maximum value at 480 nm. By reading off the absorbance values at convenient wavelength intervals, a complete spectrum can be built up.

ii.   Determination of λ_{max} by eye from the absorbance spectrum of the pigment. It is easier to measure the wavelength at which the absorbance is a certain fraction of the maximum value (e.g. 50%) and calculate the λ_{max} for the nomogram. The lower line in Fig. 3.11 represents a pigment that has an absorbance of 50% of maximum at 550 nm. The line passing through this point cuts the right-hand (λ_{max}) scale at 503 nm.

The latter operation may be performed more accurately by using the " λ_{max}-finder" (Fig. 3.12) which shows the λ_{max} values corresponding to λ_x values for A_x/A_{max} = 10, 20, ... 90% on

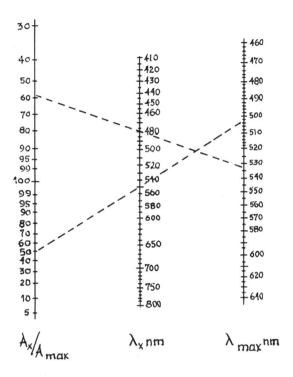

Fig. 3.11: Nomogram for the calculation of the spectra of rhodopsin pigments. The dotted lines give two examples of its use.

Upper dotted line: The absorbance at 480 nm of a rhodopsin of
λ_{max} = 533 nm is 59% of the maximum value;

Lower dotted line: A rhodopsin with an absorbance of 50% of maximum at 550 nm on the long-wave side of the peak has a λ_{max} of 503 nm.

Based on the data of Fig. 3.10.

the long-wavelength side of the absorbance maximum. The λ_x values corresponding to these percentages are measured off the spectrum, and the corresponding λ_{max} values off Fig. 3.12. These should differ by less than 2 nm. The arithmetic mean is then taken as the true λ_{max}. Since only the long-wavelength part of the spectrum is used, the method can be equally well applied to either the absolute absorbance spectrum, or the hydroxylamine difference spectrum. Caution must be exercised when using the λ_{max}-finder with the difference spectra (even those obtained in the presence of

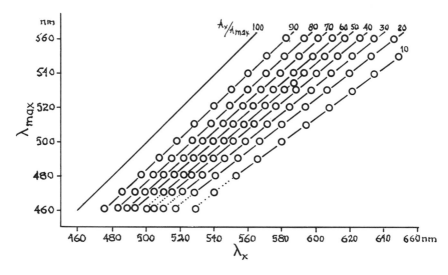

Fig. 3.12: The "λ_{max}-finder" chart for determining the exact λ_{max} of a rhodopsin from the shape of its bleaching difference spectrum. The lines relate the λ_{max} of a rhodopsin with the wavelengths of the points 10, 20, . . 100% of maximum absorbance on the long-wave side of the standard rhodopsin (Fig. 3.10). The chart is used by reading the wavelengths corresponding to 10, 20, . . 90% peak absorbance from the experimental difference spectrum, converted to 9 estimates of λ_{max} by means of the chart, and taking the mean of some or all of these as the true λ_{max}.
(After Dartnall & Lythgoe, 1965)

λ_{max} lower than 510 nm the photoproduct absorption will cause an appreciable distortion of the short-wave side of the peak away from the true nomogram shape. The curve is depressed and will therefore give λ_{max} values higher than the true one.

The Porphyropsin Nomogram

The spectra of porphyropsin pigments do not fit the Dartnall nomogram for rhodopsin. The spectrum of porphyropsin being broader than the spectrum of a rhodopsin with a corresponding λ_{max}. Based on similar principles as rhodopsin, the porphyropsin nomogram was constructed (Munz & Schwanzara, 1967; Bridges, 1967). Figures 3.13, 3.14 and 3.15 give the standard spectrum for

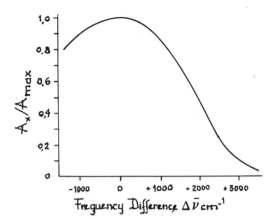

Fig. 3.13: Standard spectrum for porphyropsin pigments plotted on a wavenumber scale relative to λ_{max}. From Knowles & Dartnall, 1977)

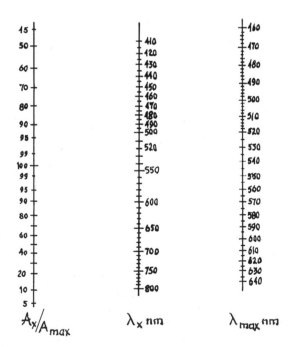

Fig. 3.14: Nomogram for the calculation of the spectra of porphyropsin, based on the data of Fig. 3.13. It is used in the same way as Fig. 3.11.

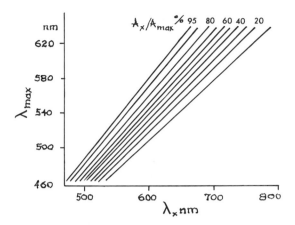

Fig. 3.15: The "λ_{max}-finder" chart for determining the exact λ_{max} of a porphyropsin from the shape of its bleaching difference spectrum. It is based on the standard spectrum of Fig. 3.13 and is used in the same way as Fig. 3.12.

porphyropsin, and the nomogram and λ_{max}-finder (based on Fig. 3.13), respectively.

Reflexion Technique

Another method for studying visual pigments, besides extracting them, is to study the reflexion properties of the visual pigments. In this technique (known as "fundus reflectometry" or "retinal densitometry"), a narrow parallel beam of light is shone into the eye to be brought to a focus on the retina, with a portion passing through the pigment epithelium. The latter absorbs most of the light, but a small portion of it is reflected, to pass once again through the receptor, through the lens, and out of the eye. As the incident light passes over the photoreceptor outer segments containing the visual pigments, lights of specific wavelengths are absorbed. Thus, if a series of wavelengths throughout the spectrum is used, less of those which are maximally absorbed will return through the pupil. The amount of reflexion at each wavelength is measured in the dark-adapted eye when there is a good concentration of pigment. The eye is then light-adapted, to bleach the pigments, and the measurements repeated. In this way the difference spectra of the living retina can be obtained. Only about 0,01 % of the incident light emerges from the eye. An ophthalmoscopic device is used to separate the emergent beam from the incident beam.

An instrument was designed by Rushton (see Hood & Rushton, 1971) to minimise the amounts of stray light, from either the bleaching or measuring source, that reach the detector (Fig. 3.16). To achieve this, paths taken by the incident and emergent beams are kept as far apart as possible, and the bleaching light is cut off by the sector-wheel while a measurement is being made. The measuring beam is also alternated with a long-wavelength moni-toring beam, which is little absorbed by the pigments in the retina, in order to compensate for slight movements of the eye and fluctuations in the light intensity. A slightly different spectrum is used by Weale (see Ripps & Weale, 1963). Here the reflexion from the subject's eye is compared to that from an artificial 'eye' acting as a monitor (Fig. 3.16). While the former instrument gives quantitative measurements at single wavelengths, the latter rapidly scans through a series of wavelengths.

The low efficiency of the reflexion means that bright measuring beams must be used, and these bleach the visual pigment to some extent. In addition, the smaller the retinal area illuminated, the greater must be the light intensity to maintain the same intensity of photons leaving the eye. Measurements are usually made on areas of the retina subtending an angle of about 5° ($\simeq$ 2 mm^2) although measurements on an area of 200 μm^2 have also been made (Weale, 1968). Despite this small area, there are a large number of photoreceptors, and if more than one type is present their individual spectra can be obtained by bleaching away the pigment in others. In practice this is difficult; first, because cone pigment regeneration is quite fast; and second, because it is impossible to select a bleaching light that will completely bleach one pigment without affecting the others. Fundus reflectometry has shown the broad spectra of scotopic pigments (cat, guinea pig, rabbit); and the narrow spectra of photic pigments from the pure cone region of the human fovea and pure cone retina of the grey squirrel. This technique has proved most useful in the study ·of human vision and has provided insights which could not have been obtained by other methods.

Microspectrophotometry (MSP)

In addition to the above techniques, visual pigments may also be measured by the technique of microspectrophotometry (MSP). This method, introduced by Caspersson (1940), combines micro-scopy and spectrophotometry. The light microscope affords the

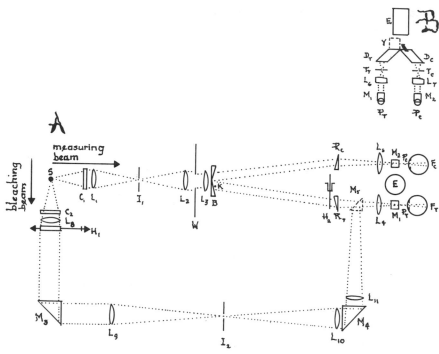

Fig. 3.16: "Fundus Reflectometry" or "Retinal Densitometry".
A Xenon-arc (S) provides the source for both measuring and
bleaching beams. The former passes sequentially through a
series of 26 interference filters mounted on a wheel (W)
rotating at about 4 rev. sec^{-1}. The beam enters the eye
through the dilated pupil (P_t), passes through the retina, is
reflected at the fundus, re-traverses the retina and emerges
through the pupil. A reflecting prism (M), collects some of the
emerging rays and directs them to a sensitive photocell (E);
the output of which is displayed on a cathode ray oscilloscope
and recorded photographically. This furnishes a complete
spectral scan of the fovea - first in the dark-adapted state and
again after it has been exposed to bleaching light (regulated by
shutter H_1) for 30 sec. For each measuring wavelength the
change in density is computed from the data displayed on the
oscilloscope. Generally a schematic eye (P_c) receives the
measuring beam alternatively with the test eye (controlled by
the position of the relay-operated shutter, H_2) and its spectral
sensitivity recorded.
c - heat absorbing filter; I - slit; B - biprism; K - small black
spot; T - small apertures; D - rhomboid prisms.
(After Weale, 1965)

identification of subcellular elements, while the determination (presence and concentration) of the visual pigments is achieved through spectrophotometry. Initially the method consisted of taking a series of photomicrographs of isolated cells at different wavelengths and analysing the relative density of the images (Denton, 1954; Denton & Wyllie, 1955; Dobrowolski et al., 1955). Further development of the MSP included the use of a photo-electric detector and automatically recording spectrophotometers with great sensitivity. This field of research blossomed in the mid 1960's and led to the introduction of several new instruments such as the dual-beam ratio-recording MSP, digital computer-controlled single-beam MSP, MSP equipped with a microscope for the determination of wavelength properties of photoreceptors, rapid scanning MSP and photon-counting MSP (see Harosi, 1981).

MSP may be classified according to cell type (vertebrate, invertebrate), method of sample preparation (single cell, multi-cell, cell fragment suspension) and orientation of cell with respect to the measuring light (transverse, axial). The most commonly used method is the transverse, single cell MSP. The advantages of this method is that the light path is well defined, there is no intervening structure, the preparation is thin and is easy to make and align with the light beam. Animals are dark-adapted for at least 12 hours prior to enucleation under dim red light or infrared illumination. The cornea and lens are removed and the entire posterior portion of the eye cup incubated in low-calcium physiological saline for about an hour at ambient temperature. This aids in the removal of sensory retina with minimum damage to the photoreceptors without affecting the pigment spectra. Small ($\simeq$ 1 mm^2) pieces of sensory retina are pulled or cut from the eye cup, teased flat and maintained in the same incubation solution between two coverslips and ringed with silicone oil.

In the photon-counting MSP (PMSP) of MacNichol (1978) the spectrum is scanned repetitively once every second (Fig. 3.17). Comparisons among the pigment spectra are made possible through a monochromater equipped with a reciprocal cam, and measurements are taken at equal frequency intervals (fresnel, one fresnel or terahertz = 10^{12} Hz, = 3×10^5 nm^{-1} = 33 wave numbers (cm^{-1}) rather than wavelength). Photoelectron counts from a number of scans are averaged at 5-fresnel intervals from 400 - 800 fresnels (750 - 355 nm). A set of 50 reference scans (blank) is first made through a clear area or fovea of the preparation. Between 3 and 20 subsequent scans through photoreceptor outer segments are averaged and referred to the blank. Optical density at each 5-fresnel interval is averaged and referred to the blank.

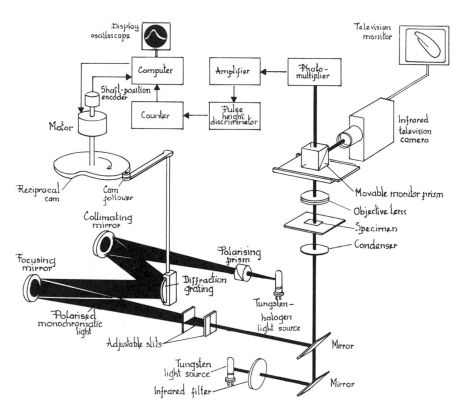

Fig. 3.17: Schematic representation of a microspectrophoto-meter. In the diagram each beam is polarised and then split into its spectral components by a diffraction grating. The wavelength of the monochromatic beam is calibrated to the position of a camshaft that controls the grating. Thus the precise wavelength of the input beam and the intensity of the output can be registered simultaneously in a computer. The pigments will bleach and lose their ability to absorb light if they are exposed to bright light. Therefore the beams passing through the specimens are held to low intensity, and the individual photons in the beam are converted into electric pulses by a photomultiplier. The pulses are then amplified from spurious signals and tallied in a counter, whose output is periodically read into a computer. To position and focus the specimens infrared illumination is used in combination with an infrared television camera and monitor.
(After Levine & MacNichol, 1982)

Preparations are placed on the microscope of the PMSP with the measuring beam $(3 - 3 \times 10^2$ μ m depending on the size of the photoreceptor outer segment under study) passing transversely through the receptors. The measuring beam bleaches an insignificant amount (little more than 10 %) of the pigment in any set of scans, no distortion of the spectral curves is introduced by bleaching. Data obtained (photon counts from sample or blank) can be used for calculation of either optical density or transmittance (Fig. 3.18). The advantage of this method of MSP is that visual pigment determinations can be made not only from single photoreceptors (Fig. 3.19), but also from the individuals of paired photoreceptors (Bowmaker et al., 1978; Levine & MacNichol, 1979; Zyznar et al., 1978). The latter has contributed to the nomenclature of paired photoreceptors (see Levine & MacNichol, 1979).

All known visual pigments utilise either retinal (Vitamin A_1) or 3, 4-dehydroretinal (Vitamin A_2) in combination with various opsins to form rhodopsins, porphyropsins and corresponding cone pigments. The retinas of some animals contain both A_1-and A_2-based pigments and it was through MSP that it was established that various rods and cones accept both chromophores equally well. MSP studies also established that vertebrate rods and cones are uniformly provided with one or a certain mixture of the homologous pair of pigments throughout the outer segment. A

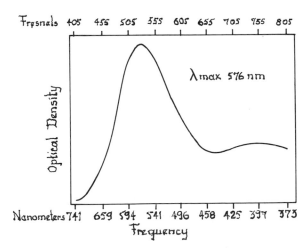

Fig. 3.18: Optical density vs frequency plot from one cell of Melanotaenia showing a λ_{max} of 576 nm. (After Levine & MacNichol, 1979)

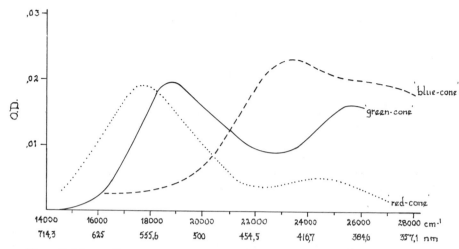

Fig. 3.19: Average optical density versus wavenumbers (cm^{-1}) spectrum of disintegrating cynomolgus (Macaca fascicularis) cone outer segments. The lower set of numbers indicate wavelengths (nm).
(From Harosi, 1982)

possible exception to this is the shift in $A_1:A_2$ ratio in some animals with changes in light conditions (Loew & Dartnall, 1976).

Difference spectra may also be obtained by MSP by measuring the absorbances of visual pigments. Values through the unbleached retina serves as the sample, the retina is then bleached and the transmission through it obtained. The absorbance of the bleached retina is then obtained from the equation:

absorbance is equal to the log of the reciprocal of transmittance.

The difference in absorbance between the bleached and unbleached retina gives the difference spectrum. Partial bleaching techniques, similar to those described for extracted pigments, may also be employed to study the homogeneity of the visual pigment if the area of illumination covers more than one visual cell.

Physiological Significance

The first event in the visual process is the absorption of light by the visual pigment contained in the outer segments of the various types of photoreceptors. Thus, the visual capacities of the animal are reflected in its visual pigments which are in turn governed by habits and habitats. This is dealt with fully under the appropriate chapters and only a brief outline will be presented here.

In general, the aldehyde base of the visual pigment gives a good indication of the environment. Terresterial and marine animals tend to have Vitamin A_1 (retinal$_1$) based pigments, while freshwater animals have Vitamin A_2 (retinal$_2$) based pigments. In addition, visual pigment changes (retinal$_1$ to retinal$_2$ and vice versa) are also noted when the animal changes its habitat during its life cycle from salt to freshwater (catadromous); from fresh to salt water (anadromous); or from freshwater to land (e.g. terresterial amphibia). A further interesting point is illustrated in species adapted for aquatic and terresterial vision at the same time (e.g. bullfrog, four-eyed fish). In these animals the visual pigments in the ventral retina (used for aerial vision) is retinal$_1$- based, while the dorsal retina (used for aquatic vision) is retinal$_2$-based.

Visual pigments also reflect the spectral qualities of the environment as exemplified in the aquatic media. Besides depth, penetration of light into water is influenced by suspended and dissolved particles. Only the high energy short wavelength lights can penetrate to any great extent. Thus, animals inhabiting deep waters generally have visual pigments with the spectra shifted to shorter wavelengths. Exceptions to this general rule are usually due to light emitting from bioluminescent organisms found in the vicinity. In clear, shallow waters the absorption maxima of the pigment is shifted to longer wavelengths (500 nm - marine; 525 nm - freshwater). In coloured or turbid waters the maxima tend to correspond to the transmission spectra of these waters and in turbid waters they shift towards longer (e.g. 535 nm) wavelengths.

4

ACCOMMODATION

All eyes have to solve the problem of imaging successfully objects at different distances, i.e. they have to exercise the power of accommodation.

In order to focus objects clearly the image has to fall on the retina, i.e. the rays of light have to converge on the photoreceptor cell layer of the retina. The refractive indices of the cornea, aqueous humour and vitreous body approximate that of water (1,33), while the material of the crystalline lens has an effective refractive index ranging from 1,42 - 1,69. Thus, in aquatic vertebrates the cornea is practically powerless in refracting light because its refractive index is similar to that of the environment; the lens therefore provides the refraction necessary for adequate image formation. Terresterial vertebrates, on the other hand, depend largely on the cornea for image formation, the lens merely supplementing the power of the cornea. In vertebrates which are highly developed visually the lens also provides fine focussing control.

Parallel rays of light (i.e. rays of light from a distant object) entering the eye of a subject with normal vision (emmetropia) are brought to focus on the retina when its accommodation is relaxed (Fig. 4.1). However, if the subject is myopic (short-sighted), as a result of the eyeball being too long, parallel rays of light are brought to focus in front of the retina (Fig. 4.1); while in the case of a hypermetropic (long-sighted) subject, where the eyeball is too short, parallel rays are brought to focus behind the retina (Fig. 4.1). The refractive error of a hypermetrope or myope can be corrected by placing, respectively, converging or diverging lenses in front of the subject's eye.

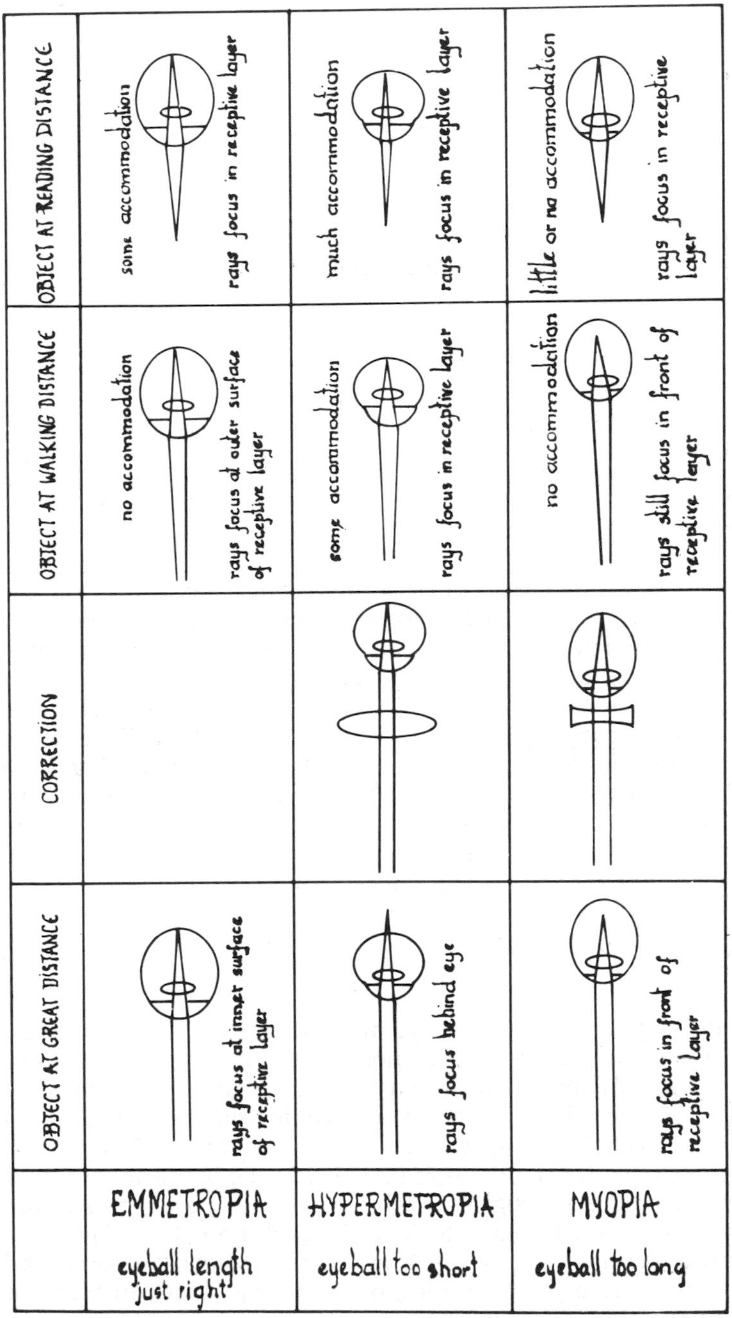

	OBJECT AT GREAT DISTANCE	CORRECTION	OBJECT AT WALKING DISTANCE	OBJECT AT READING DISTANCE
EMMETROPIA eyeball length just right	rays focus at inner surface of receptive layer		no accommodation — rays focus at outer surface of receptive layer	some accommodation — rays focus in receptive layer
HYPERMETROPIA eyeball too short	rays focus behind eye		some accommodation — rays focus in receptive layer	much accommodation — rays focus in receptive layer
MYOPIA eyeball too long	rays focus in front of receptive layer		no accommodation — rays still focus in front of receptive layer	little or no accommodation — rays focus in receptive layer

Fig. 4.1: Defects in vision due to the size of the eye ball.
(After Walls, 1942)

In ophthalmology, the power of a lens (in dioptres) is the reciprocal of its focal length in metres. Degrees of myopia and hypermetropia are usually expressed in terms of the number of dioptres of the lens necessary to give normal vision. Thus a myopic eye which needs a concave lens of 4 dioptres (focal length of 0,25 metres) would be said to have 4 dioptres of myopia. Accommodation can also be expressed in similar terms. For example, a human eye with normal vision can focus distant objects when it is relaxed, and in order to see clearly an object at 0,2 metres it will have to increase the power of the lens by 5 (1/0,2) dioptres. This is called exercising 5 dioptres of accommodation. A hypermetrope who ordinarily has to accommodate by, for example, 1 dioptre in order to see distant objects must increase his accommodation by the same 5 dioptres to see clearly at 0,2 metres. Thus, he has to accommodate a total of 6 dioptres. The normal human eye of a young adult is capable of exercising about 10 dioptres of accommodation (i.e. ∞ to 0,1 metres), but this power of accommodation gradually diminishes steadily throughout life until the condition of presbyopia (the inability to accommodate close objects) is established at around the age of 40 years or more. In this case, except for the more myopic, reading glasses are a necessity.

In addition to the above, a refractive error may arise when the power of the eye is not well matched to its axial length. It may happen that the curvature of the refracting surfaces of the eye are different along different meridians. This results in the focal length of the eye being different in different meridional planes (i.e. in different planes through the visual axis of the eye). If the shortest and longest focal lengths occur in meridional planes that are at right angles to each other, and if the focal length changes smoothly between these values then the subject is said to have regular astigmatism. This error can be corrected by placing a cylindrical lens of the correct power with the axis at such an angle so as to equalise the focal lengths in the different meridional planes. If a spherical correction is also required it is usually formed on one side of the lens while the cylindrical surface is formed on the other. Irregular astigmatism exists when the corneal surface becomes irregularly distorted, due for example to healed ulceration. In this case, the only means of correction is a 'contact' lens which effectively replaces the irregular corneal surface by an optically regular one.

The normal eyes of many animals are hypermetropic if their objects of interest tend to be at great distances; while others, owing to their particular habitat or other reasons have no cause or possibility of examining distant objects, may be normally myopic.

Not all animals are capable of exercising accommodation. Some have eyes which make it unnecessary - the lens may have a great depth of focus or the outer segments of the visual cells which receive the light stimulus may be unusually long or banked. While others, especially small mammals, have such poor vision to begin with that fine adjustments are simply not worth it. In general, only eyes organised for day-light vision and high resolution need a mechanism of accommodation to compensate for appreciable variations in object distances.

The actual mechanism of accommodation differs in the different orders of vertebrates (Fig. 4.2). Although most accom-

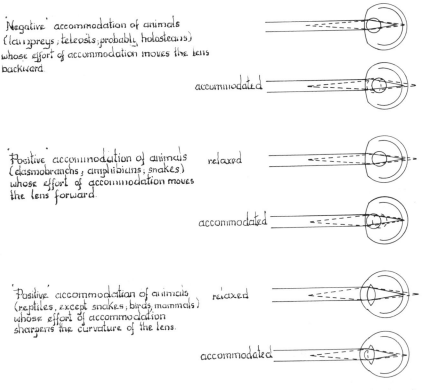

Fig. 4.2: Diagrammatic representation of general methods of accommodation - lens movement (forward or backward) and change in lens curvature - found in vertebrates.
—————   rays from distant objects
- - - -   rays from near objects

modative systems are linked to the lens (movement or deformation), nevertheless, the ability to change the power of the cornea also exists. These methods of accommodation are termed dynamic. In addition, there is static or inactive accommodation, here the structure of the eye and the retina may eliminate the need for adjustments of the refracting surfaces. However, as it is difficult, without considerable repetition, to seperate one type of accommodation from the other the different aspects of accommodation will be examined under the major vertebrate taxonomic headings.

Fishes

The primary optical difference between aquatic and terresterial vertebrates is that in the eye of the latter the cornea is the major refracting medium, while in the former the crystalline lens acts as the refractive element. In addition to a high refractive index ($\simeq$ 1,654), the crystalline lens of fishes is usually firm and spherical in shape; this suggests that lens movement (Fig. 4.3), rather than deformation, would be the most apt means of accommodation.

Active Accommodation

The eye of teleosts is thought to be myopic in the accommodated state because the restricted distance that light travels in water would favour the visibility of near objects. Contraction of the intra-ocular muscle, retractor lentis or campanulae, moves the lens sideways and backwards towards the retina, thus accommodating for distant vision. There has, however, been some contradiction to the suggestion that fish eyes are myopic. Opponents of this suggestion reported a predominance of hypermetropia in a number of freshwater fishes. They suggest that contraction of ciliary muscle fibres, having no direct or indirect articulation with the lens, is responsible for the elongation of the axial length of the eye, thus accommodating the eye for distant vision.

Although recent studies support the former suggestion (that the eyes of teleosts are myopic) there is disagreement concerning the direction of accommodative lens movement, and variation in the direction of accommodation among species has been emphasised. While in the majority of the species studied the main accommodative lens movement is found close to the pupil plane (e.g. the yellow perch, Perca flavescens; the northern rock bass, Ambloplites rupestris rupestris), in others the principal direction of

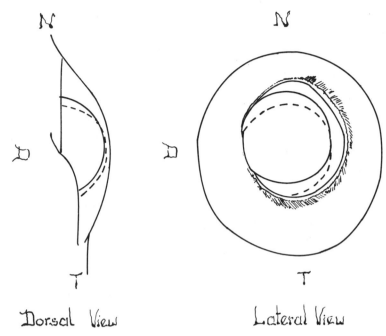

Dorsal View   Lateral View

Fig. 4.3:   Diagrammatic representation of the nasal (N) to temporal (T) lens movement in the right eye of bluegill (Lepomis macrochirus, Perciformes). D - dorsal.
(After Somiya & Tamura, 1973)

lens motion is along the pupil axis (e.g. the goldfish, Carassius auratus; the common white sucker, Catostomus commersonni). The former group has the more 'visual' feeding habits and exhibit larger amounts of lens movement (equivalent to 20 dioptres or more). In addition, lens motion in the pupil plane is usually associated with an indented pupil margin thus creating a lensless or aphakic space. Circumstantial evidence suggests that the size and orientation of this space is related to the magnitude and direction of accommodation.

Very little information has been paid to the group of non-teleost fishes, and often the information available is either contradictory or in need of further verification.

Lampreys and hagfishes belong to the most primitive vertebrate class, the Agnatha. The burrowing parasitic behaviour of hagfishes coincides with an advanced level of ocular degeneration, but, in the lamprey the eye is well developed.

Early studies on the European lamprey (Lampetra fluviatilis) by Franz suggest that the eye of this lamprey can accommodate in three different ways. Firstly, the contraction of an extra-ocular muscle, the cornealis, flattens the spectacle and cornea, thus pushing the lens toward the retina thereby providing accommodation for distant objects - eye myopic at rest. Secondly, contraction of all six extra-ocular muscles involved in eye movement results in the elongation of the optic axis and an increase in the lens to retina distance - accommodation for distant vision, eye hypermetropic. Thirdly, unilateral stimulation of the head muscles produces refractive changes toward myopia when the head is bent toward the observer and hypermetropia when it is bent in the opposite direction. These studies, however, have still to be verified. Retinoscopic refractive state measurements on the sea lamprey (Petromyzon marinus) indicate that the eye of this lamprey shows high levels of hypermetropia (≃ 17 dioptres) and that there is only a slight reduction (≃ 3 dioptres) at the level of electrical stimulation capable of producing contraction of muscles over the head of the animal. Furthermore, the absence of the cornealis muscle negates the first method of accommodation suggested by Franz. These negative results, however, do not prove that all lampreys are incapable of accommodation, especially as different species are involved. The parasitic behaviour of most adult lampreys does not point to the need for a large accommodative ability.

Elasmobranchs (cartilagenous fishes: sharks, rays and skates) are known to have eyes which are hypermetropic at rest. However, the fact that light travels through a limited distance in water, and that the eye of most elasmobranchs do not accommodate questions the practicality for hypermetropism. The sharks (the nurse shark, Ginglymostoma cirratum, and the sand bar shark, Carcharinus milberti), accommodate by contraction of the protactor lentis muscle; while the spiny dogfish (Squalus acanthias) and the lemon shark (Negaprion brevirostris) do not accommodate. The blunt-nosed stingray (Dasyatis sayi) also exhibits active accommodation. The refractive state is altered in the direction of myopia (or less hypermetropia) as the target distance is decreased.

References to chondrosteans and holosteans are again scanty. Although no accommodation could be induced electrically in chondrosteans, such as the sturgeon (Acipenser fulvescens), a muscle similar to the protactor lentis muscle of the elasmobranchs was present. In holosteans (the genera Amia and Lepisosteus) a muscle resembling the retractor lentis of teleosts in microscopial morphology and location is present, and these fishes exhibit lens movement along the pupil axis.

Inactive Accommodation

Ramp Retina

'Ramp' retina refers to a static accommodation mechanism which is the result of asymmetry of the eye about the lens (Fig. 4.4); the axial length of the eyeball changes continuously in a vertical meridian. Fishes such as the flatfishes, skates and rays employ this ocular asymmetry as a means of accommodation. The head or the eye is moved so as to produce a new visual axis that includes a longer lens to retina distance for viewing near objects. In addition to the retina, other means of dynamic accommodation may also be present as observed in the bluntnose stingray (Dasyatis sayi) and the gulf flounder (Paralichthys albigutta).

Multiple Optic Axis

A typical example of a fish employing this method of accommodation is the four-eyed fish (Anableps anableps). In this, and related species, the dorsal half of each eye is exposed to air, while the nasal and temporal extensions of the iris create a double

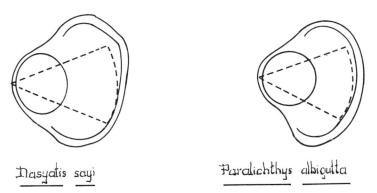

Dasyatis sayi   Paralichthys albigutta

Fig. 4.4: Vertical section through the eye of a ray (Dasyatis sayi) and a flounder (Paralichthys albigutta) showing how the retina forms a "ramp" - the axial length of the eyeball changes continuously in the vertical meridian.
(After Sivak, 1980)

pupil (Fig. 4.5). In contrast to the usual spherical lens, the lens of Anableps is oval, thus providing two axes. The long axis corresponds to the ventral axis (aquatic) and the short axis corresponds to the dorsal axis (aerial) (Fig. 4.5). The difference in the refractive state measured through the two pupils while the dorsal half of the cornea is in air and the ventral half is in water confirms that the variation in lens shape compensates for the presence and absence of a corneal refractive contribution. The retina too is divided into dorsal (aquatic) and ventral (aerial) portions, and it has been demonstrated that the optic nerve fibres from the two parts of the retina project separately to the optic tectum.

Corneal Facets (Flattened Cornea)

Flat, corneal facets may also be employed to deal with aerial-aquatic vision. In the Atlantic flying fish (Cypselurus

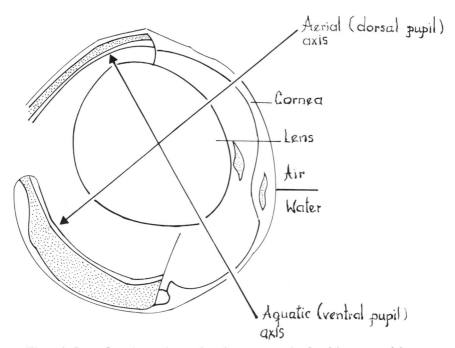

Fig. 4.5: Section through the eye of Anableps anableps showing the multiple optic axis method of accommodation used by this fish.

heterurus) the cornea is composed of three flat triangular facets that meet in the centre. As little or no light is refracted by the cornea in either medium there is little difference between the aerial and aquatic images. Faceted corneas were also observed in two teleosts of the family Clinidae, Dialommus fuscus and Mnierpes macrocephalus; which occupy an intertidal habitat and thus require amphibious visual capabilities.

Receptor Length, Banked Receptors and Depth of Focus

These characteristics are usually associated with increase in retinal sensitivity as it is generally assumed that light striking the photoreceptor outer segments is required to invoke the visual impulse. Nevertheless increase in the length of the outer segments of the photoreceptors, and banked receptors may also provide a means of static accommodation as they provide for changes in focal depth.

Amphibians

The phylogenetic bridge between aquatic and terresterial vertebrate life is represented by the amphibians, and as such they are faced with the problem of having to see both in water and in air. The optical appearance of the eye of the larval forms is essentially similar to that of the teleost fishes while the eye of the adult approaches that of the higher terresterial forms. Although amphibians have been used extensively for the study of the anatomy, physiology and chemistry of vision, the optical character-istics of the amphibian eye have been largely ignored.

A recent study (du Pont & de Groot, 1976) confirms that although the lens of the adult frog (Rana esculenta) is somewhat flattened it is unlikely to change its shape because of its firmness, thus lens movement is suggested (Fig. 4.6). Its equivalent refractive index of 1,65 is similar to that found in teleost fishes, however, the eye of the frog is emmetropic in air, but becomes highly hypermetropic in water as the power of the cornea is somewhat eliminated. In water, the eye is covered by the nictitating membrane, but as the refractive index of this membrane and the cornea are similar, the eye remains hypermetropic. However, if a thin film of air is trapped between the nictitating membrane and the cornea the eye would remain as it is in air. In addition, smooth muscle cells have been noted in the amphibian choroid and the possibility that these muscles may play a role in active accommodation cannot be ruled out (Walls, 1942).

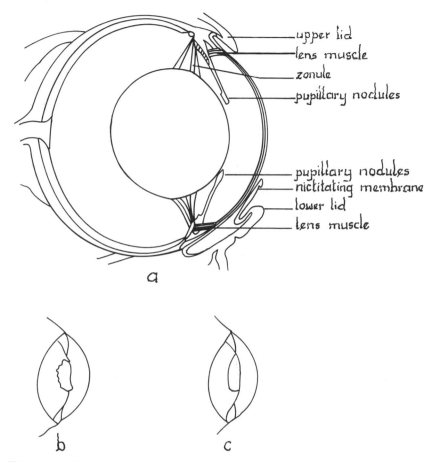

Fig. 4.6: The amphibian eye and its accommodation.
a.   Vertical section of an anuran eye, based mainly on Rana
        pipiens
b, c   Anterior segment of Bufo sp in relaxation and accom-
        modation, respectively. Note the forward movement of
        the lens.
(After Walls, 1942).

        Unfortunately the question of accommodation in larval
amphibians has never received direct attention. Furthermore,
accommodation in amphibians should not be directed solely to frogs
and toads. It is apparent that the adult frog (R. esculenta) and
salamander (Salamander salamandra) have a terresterial visual

system - both are emmetropic in air and possess somewhat flattened lenses. In contrast, the larval form of S. salamandra and Triturus cristatus (a newt, the adult of which exhibits both terresterial and aquatic behaviour) have eyes with aquatic characteristics - both are emmetropic in water and possess spherical lenses. The newt is also known to be strongly myopic in air.

Reptiles and Birds

.   Reptiles and birds exhibit essentially similar accommodative mechanisms, this may reflect the phylogenetic affinity between these two vertebrate classes. Basically the focal power of the eye is varied by changes in the shape of the crystalline lens brought about by the action of the powerful, striated ciliary muscle. In addition, the ciliary body is in direct contact with the lens. Thus the anterior and inward movement of the ciliary body in response to ciliary muscle contraction results in equatorial pressure on the lens which then, because of physical constraints on the anterior peripherical and posterior lens surfaces by the iris and the vitreous humour, result in the central surface of the lens being squeezed out towards the cornea. In addition to lens deformation, corneal accommodation also exists. This is especially true in birds.

The major emphasis of recent research dealing with accommodation in reptiles and birds have been directed towards the amphibious species. These vertebrates must possess adequate mechanisms for maintaining adequate visual optics in both air and in water. It has been suggested that the crystalline power of the lens may have great refractive power and is relatively soft. This is coupled to the lens deforming power of the ciliary muscle which may be assisted by the sphincter muscle of the iris.

Reptiles

The eye of aquatic turtles of the genus Emys (e.g. E. orbicularis), is known to be emmetropic both in air and in water. This is achieved presumably through accommodation rendered by the iris (Fig. 4.7). Other turtles, however, differ. The eye of the marine turtle (Chelonia mydas), which is extremely myopic in air, has typical aquatic characteristics - a more spherical lens and the existence of a shallow anterior chamber. In addition, it lacks direct contact between the ciliary processes and the lens, as well as the large iris sphincter. The eye of the land tortoise (Gopherus polyphemus), on the other hand, is typically terresterial and the refractive neutralisation of the cornea in water (eye hypermetropic

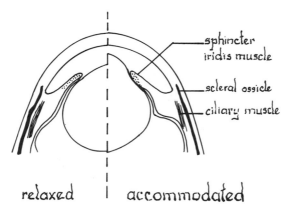

Fig. 4.7:   Accommodation in the turtle, Emys orbicularis, through lens deformation. The lens is extremely soft and its deformation is effected through the action of the ciliary muscles and the sphincter iridis. During accommodation the lens is squeezed equatorially.
(After Walls, 1942)

in water) is made up by its great accommodative ability.

Snakes differ in their mode of accommodation; lens movement rather than deformation is involved (Fig. 4.8). A study (Sivak, 1977) of three diurnal snake species showed that the lens plays a greater refractive role than it does in a diurnal lizard (e.g. Iguana iguana) and that the refractive loss of the cornea is replaced by the spectacle itself. However, if the size of the spectacle is much larger than the eye, the contribution of the spectacle would be negligible. In addition, the small size of the eyes in these species suggests that the eye functions as a light detector and does not perform any important visual task.

Birds

Active Accommodation

It is generally accepted that the principal mode of accommodation in birds involves changes in lens curvature brought about by the apparatus consisting of a striated ciliary muscle, ciliary processes, annular pad, and scleral ossicles (Fig. 4.9). The power of accommodation of birds is probably greater than that of any other vertebrates, and this is especially true of aquatic birds which can see as well under water as they can in air.

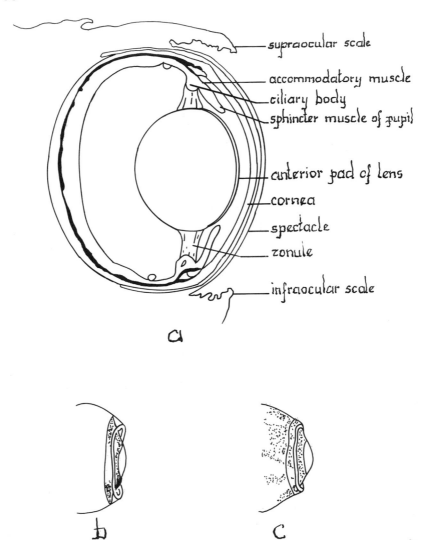

Fig. 4.8: The ophidian eye and its accommodation.
a.   Vertical section of the eye of the European grass snake
      Natrix natrix.
b, c. Anterior segment of Coluber æsculapii in relaxation and
      accommodation, respectively, the dome of the cornea
      has been cut away to show the method of accom-
      modation.   Note the forward movement of the lens and
      the decrease of the eyeball diameter at limbus (c).
(After Walls, 1942)

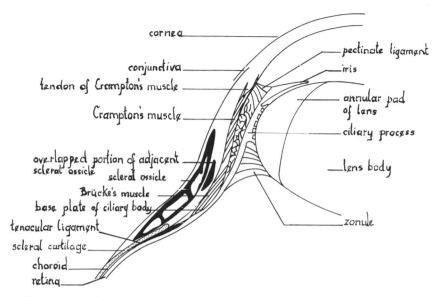

Fig. 4.9: Semi-diagrammatic representation of the accom-
modatory apparatus of birds based on the situation in hawks.

In species exercising corneal accommodation, the ciliary
muscle is divided into two portions - Crampton's muscle responsible
for altering corneal curvature, and Brücke's muscle responsible for
altering lens curvature.   The strongest support for corneal
accommodation is provided by Gundlach et al. (1945). Using a
modified ophthalmometer to measure the corneal curvature of the
pigeon's eye, they found that the pigeon could achieve 17 dioptres
by corneal accommodation. In recent years, however, doubts have
arisen over this form of accommodation.   In the owl (Bubo
virginiansus), the presence of the large Crampton's muscle is not
associated with corneal accommodation. Nevertheless, the eyes of
birds such as the hawk and eagle are known to possess superior
resolving power (2 - 3 times that of the human eye), and as corneal
accommodation is usually considered to supplement lens effects
future studies on species with superior acuity might prove
profitable.

The possibility that the iris may contribute to an exaggerated
accommodative ability has been discussed in relation to the
amphibious reptiles. Many avian species also depend on the aquatic
environment for food and as such require amphibious vision.

Birds (e.g. the cormorant, Phalacrocorax auritus; the black guillemot, Cepphus grylle; the hooded merganser, Mergus cucullatus; and penguins) which have to pursue their prey under water are emmetropic, or very nearly so, both in air and in water. Histological studies have shown that the accommodated eye exhibits a central, anterior lens bulge of very short radius of curvature; and from the pupillary position of the bulge it is clear that the iris, rather than the ciliary body, is responsible for accommodation (Fig. 4.10).

Pelicans (Pelecanus occidentalis) which plunge and dive for fish on a hit and miss basis; gulls (Larus argentatus) which scavenge for food at the water surface, and the common mallard (Anas platyrhynchos) which feed on vegetable are emmetropic in air, but become extremely hypermetropic in water. These birds do not show histological evidence of the contribution of the iris in accommodation.

Inactive Accommodation

Nictitating Membrane

The possibility that the nictitating membrane of the bird eye may contribute to altering the refractive power of the eye was first suggested in 1912. It was noted that in diving ducks (Mergus

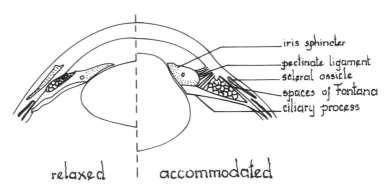

Fig. 4.10:   Accommodation in amphibious birds, e.g. Phalacrocorax sp.   Note the action of the powerful iris sphincter, and that in the accommodated state the fibres of the pectinate ligament are taut and that the spaces of Fontana, behind them, have become dilated by the action of the iris.   (After Walls, 1942)

merganser) and loons (Gavia lumme) there is a central, transparent window of high refractive index which would help compensate for the neutralising effect of water on the cornea. Recent studies (Sivak, 1980) have disputed this proposal, and it has been suggested that unless an example of a membrane with an obviously different shape (central bulge of short radius of curvature and high refractive index, or flattened membrane capable of trapping air between it and the cornea) can be shown (Fig. 4.11) the refractive role of the nictitating membrane seems doubtful (Fig. 4.12).

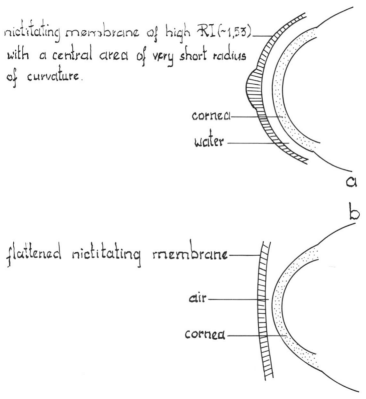

Fig. 4.11: Schematic representations of two hypothetical possibilities. The first (a) is based on the existence of a nictitating membrane of high refractive index (RI) with a central area of very short radius of curvature. The second (b) is based on the existence of a flattened nictitating membrane which traps air between it and the cornea, as in a diver's goggle. Neither case is known to exist in nature. (From Sivak et al., 1978)

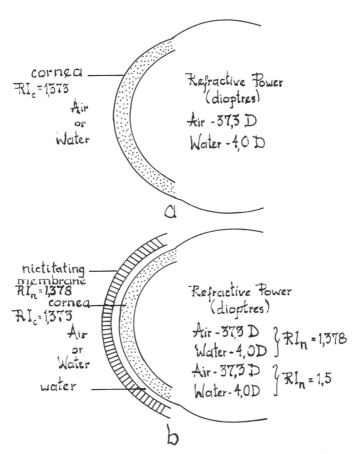

Fig. 4.12:   Refractive power of the anterior surface of a
hypothetical bird in air and in water, and with (a) and without
(b) the nictitating membrane in place.   If the nictitating
membrane has parallel sides and a curvature equal to that of
the cornea then the refractive situation is unchanged irre-
spective of the refractive index of the membrane (e.g. RI_n =
1,378 or 1,5; b).   Refractive indices of the cornea (RL_c =
1,373) and nictitating membrane (RI_n = 1,378) are those of the
common mallard.
(After Sivak et al., 1978)

Flattened Cornea

The optical effect of moving from air to water (and vice versa) is minimised by the existence of a relatively flat cornea. Penguins, which are aquatic feeders, are found to have radii of curvature of the cornea 25 - 30% greater than that of the whole eye. The fact that corneal curvature is one of the principal factors governing the size of the visual field suggests that penguins have paid for their amphibious adaptation with a loss of field size in air.

Multiple Optic Axis

It has been suggested (Kolmer, 1924) that the eye of birds such as the kingfisher (Alcedo attis attis) may be capable of aerial-aquatic vision in a manner similar to the four-eyed fish (Anableps anableps). Although the presence of two foveas, oval lens and better developed ciliary muscle on the nasal side have been put forward in support of this proposal, further study on the eye of the kingfisher is still required.

Mammals

Active Accommodation

It is commonly assumed that human accommodative mechanism (Fig. 4.13) is representative of all mammals having accommodative abilities. However, the study of accommodation in mammals (other than humans) has been grossly neglected and the results are often contradictory. Accordingly, it has been reported that only primates are capable of accommodative ranges found in young humans (about 10 dioptres). Then, there are reports that the cat is able to accommodate, by lens movement, from 2 - 15 dioptres. Rabbits and rats, on the other hand, are unable to accommodate. Furthermore, it is generally thought that the eye of small mammals and nocturnal mammals are hypermetropic; the latter merely signifying an indifference to the need for optical quality. While the otter (e.g. Amblonyx cineria cineria), an amphibious mammal, is thought to compensate for the refractive loss of the cornea in water by means of an iris accommodative mechanism similar to that found in amphibious reptiles and birds.

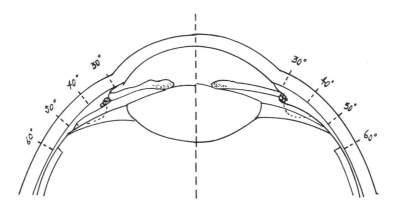

Fig. 4.13: Mammalian (human) accommodation. Diagram of
the anterior part of the human eye and changes due to
accommodation; by reference to the angular scales, the
movements of the various parts can be discerned. Note that
the contraction of both the radial and circumferential portions
of the ciliary muscle has stretched forward the smooth
orbicular region of the ciliary body (to which most of the
zonule fibres attach) and has bunched up the corneal region
(bearing the ciliary processes, whose profiles are indicated by
the dotted lines). The relaxation of the zonule fibres has
permitted the elastic lens capsule to mold a bulge of sharpened
curvature on the anterior surface of the lens. Note also that
the sphincter muscle of the iris has contracted, closing down
the pupil in its "accommodation reflex".
(After Walls, 1942)

Inactive Accommodation

Flattened Cornea and/or Stenopeic Pupil

    Mammals, such as the seal, require amphibious vision. In
water light is brought to focus in the eye of the seal (e.g. the harp
seal, Phagophilus groenlandicus; the Weddell seal, Leptonychotes
weddelli; the harbour seal, Phoca vitulina) by a nearly spherical
lens. In air, the refractive effect of the cornea is minimised due to
the cornea being flattened along the vertical margin and the
contraction of the pupil into a vertical slit in air (it is dilated and
rounded in water). The pupil also acts as a stenopeic slit to
increase the depth of focus.

Ramp Retina

A 'ramp' retina, though less exaggerated than that found in rays, is found in the horse. In this type of eye (see Fig. 4.4) distant objects are focussed on the inferior part of the retina which is nearer to the lens and nearer objects on the superior part, with a smooth transition between them.   The horse has no means of changing the focal length of its lens, but can change the position of the image within the retina by tilting its head. An eye with a ramp retina is set to a distant focus for objects overhead and to a near one for objects underneath.   This, however, has been contested by Sivak and Allen (1975).

Receptor Structure

Increase in the length, or the effective length of the visual cells, although primarily a means of increasing sensitivity may have an incidental effect in partially obviating accommodation.   The Megachiroptera (great fruit bats or flying foxes) have a unique retinal structure.   It has a choroidal papillae whose internal contours provide an undulating surface over which are arranged the photoreceptors (Fig. 4.14). One of the functions attributed to the papillae is that it provides multiple focal planes, thereby

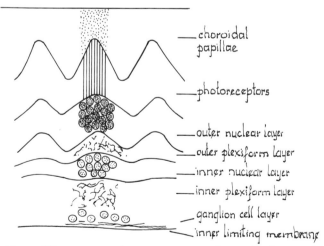

Fig. 4.14:   Diagrammatic representation of the retina of Pteropus giganteus showing the choroidal papillae which places the visual cells at various levels.
(After Howland, 1983)

eliminating the need for active accommodation (Walls, 1942). However, an active accommodative mechanism was found in the flying fox (Pteropus giganteus) (Howland, 1983).

Multiple Optic Paths

The fact that the refractive index of the vertebrate lens decreases from the centre to the periphery has been referred to as a factor reducing spherical aberration of the eye. It has been suggested that the dolphin lens is over-corrected for spherical aberration to the extent that the index of the periphery is sufficiently reduced to neutralise the refractive contribution of the cornea in air (Rivamonte, 1976). A visual axis coinciding with the centre of the lens is used in water, whereas a peripheral axis is used in air. This theory has still to be verified.

5

ADAPTATIONS TO LIGHT AND DIMNESS

The earth receives, almost exclusively, radiation from the sun; the spectrum of which encompasses ultraviolet to infrared radiation (Fig. 5.1). Within this, only a narrow region of the continuum (visible light) is detectable by the eyes of living organisms. The visible light, defined in terms of human sensitivity, ranges from about 400 nm (violet) to 700 nm (red) (Fig. 5.1). To the human, the sunlight's spectral composition appears white. This natural source of illumination can vary in intensities by a factor of 10^{15} from a clear, bright, sunny day to a dark, moonless night (Table 3). Thus to function efficiently the eye must 'adapt' to the incident light; it must be able to capture the few photons available in darkness and to protect itself in bright light when bleaching of the visual pigments can become a problem. Remarkably, the human visual system can operate over most of this range (Table 5.1). The ability to adapt to different light intensities is required not only during the gradual change from day to night and vice versa, but also during the much faster changes associated with movements between areas of different light intensities. When we leave a brightly lit area and enter a darkened area we experience temporary 'blindness' until our vision improves. This increase in visual sensitivity with time is called dark-adaptation. Under reverse conditions (entering a brightly lit area from a darkened one) our eyes must adjust to the excess light. This loss of sensitivity to increased ambient light intensities is termed light-adaptation.

Several mechanisms of light- and dark-adaptation are employed by the visual system. A particular species may adopt a single mechanism or a combination of mechanisms. These mechanisms operate at different levels in the visual system and

95

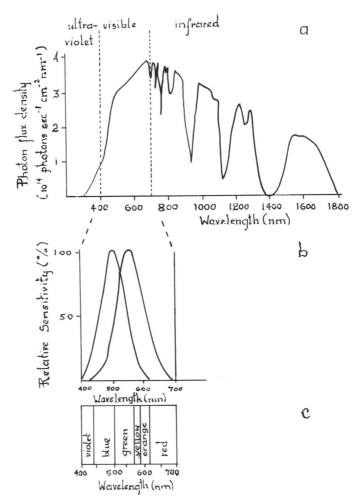

Fig. 5.1: (a) Spectral distribution of sunlight as measured on the surface of the earth on a cloudless day with the sun's elevation 30° above the horizon. Total incident radiation within the visible range (400 -700 nm) is about 10^{17} photons $cm^{-2}sec^{-1}$. (b) Spectral sensitivity of the normal human eye when ambient light intensities are dim (dark-adapted eye or scotopic vision) or bright (light-adapted eye or photopic vision). (c) Distribution of colours within the visible spectrum as seen by man.
(**a** - after Seliger, 1977; **b, c** - after LeGrand, 1957)

Table 5.1: Range of light intensities naturally encountered and the range of human vision (After Fein & Szuts, 1982)

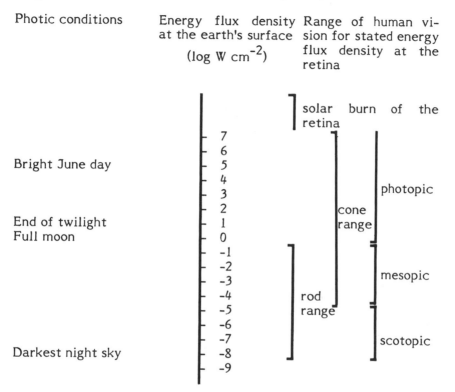

Photic conditions	Energy flux density at the earth's surface (log W cm^{-2})	Range of human vision for stated energy flux density at the retina
	7	solar burn of the retina
Bright June day	6	
	5	
	4	
	3	photopic
	2	
End of twilight	1	cone range
Full moon	0	
	-1	
	-2	
	-3	mesopic
	-4	
	-5	rod range
	-6	
	-7	scotopic
Darkest night sky	-8	
	-9	

may be divided into three classes:-
1. Regulation of light reaching the visual pigment in the photoreceptors;
2. Absorption by the visual pigment;
3. Neural processing.

Regulation of Light Reaching the Visual Pigment

The regulation of the amount of light entering the eye and reaching the photosensitive outer segments may be brought about through the control of pupil size or movements within the retina itself.

Pupil Size

The most obvious manner in which the eye can regulate the amount of light reaching the retina is to control the quantity of light entering it - pupil regulation. Round pupils cannot close completely and the difference between the amount of light entering the eye when the pupil is fully opened and 'closed' is about 1 log unit (1,2 log units for the human pupil). Slit pupils, common in non-basking nocturnal reptiles and nocturnal mammals, can reduce their effective apertures to almost zero. Besides round and slit pupils, more elaborate pupil configurations are also present (see Chapter 6). These are present in shallow-living aquatic animals, particularly bottom-living species (e.g. flat fishes, rays). Here the dorsal margin of the iris develops into a flap which overlaps all but the ventral rim of the pupil. In its more elaborate form the flap forms a fringe, thereby forming a series of little pupils in a semi-circle around the ventral margin of the pupil (e.g. ray; see Chapter 6).

The change in pupil size in mammals in response to varying intensities is temporary, thus permitting the other slower adaptive processes in the retina (e.g. retinomotor movements) to adjust to the level of the light intensity. Pupil dilation/contraction may be rapid (1 - 2 seconds; e.g. birds, reptiles, mammals) or slow (2 - 3 minutes; e.g. elasmobranchs). It is interesting to note that the rapid pupil movements observed in birds are related not to adaptations to different light intensities, but rather to accommodation and the emotional state of the bird.

Retinomotor (Photomechanical) Movements

The positional changes of photoreceptors (rods and cones) and the melanin granules within the pigment epithelial cells (RPE) of the retina in response to different levels of illumination are collectively known as retinomotor or photomechanical movements. Phylogenetically these movements appear to be older than pupillary movements, and are observed in fishes, amphibians and birds. Incidentally, photomechanical movements were studied, independently by Boll and Kühne as early as 1877. Since then, this phenomenon has been re-examined and reviewed several times (see Ali, 1971, 1975).

Photomechanical movements are initiated by photoactivated rhodopsin. This is based on experimental evidence which indicates that the action spectrum for pigment migration is matched by the absorption of rhodopsin and not that of melanin (Ali & Crouzy,

1968; Liebman et al., 1969). Apparently, photoactivation of rhodopsin must precede photomechanical movements, however, the connexion between the two is unknown. In some species, photomechanical movements appear to be controlled by an endogenous rhythm. In these species ambient illumination affects retinal movements, however, full expression of the components involved are seen only when exogenous conditions are synchronised to the internal circadian rhythm. Other factors which may influence photomechanical movements include temperature, oxygen tension (in fish) and emotional disturbance.

Photomechanical movements may involve the movement of one or both photoreceptors (rods and cones) and/or migration of the screening pigment (melanin) granules of the retina (Fig. 5.2)

Photoreceptor Movement

In vertebrates, photoreceptor movement is expressed through the radial contraction and elongation of the myoid - the contractile region which connects the ellipsoid to the nucleus. The molecular mechanism of photoreceptor movement is thought to be based on the contractility of the cytoskeletal elements - microfilaments (actin) and microtubules (Anctil et al., 1980; Burnside, 1978; Couillard, 1975; Ferrero et al., 1979; O'Connor & Burnside, 1981; Warren & Burnside, 1978) (Fig. 5.3). One or both sets of photoreceptors may be involved. Thus, in the trout both rods and cones respond to illumination, while in the walleye and common catfish the cones are static. Light-adaptation initiates elongation of rods and contraction of cones, while dark-adaptation initiates the reverse (Fig. 5.2).

Screening Pigment Movement

In vertebrate retinas screening pigments are found within the pigment epithelium (except in albinos). These pigment granules may be stationary or mobile. When mobile, pigment granules migrate, in response to light, into the apical processes of the epithelial cells, thereby shrouding the outer segments of the rods which elongate in light. In darkness, the pigment granules re-aggregates within the basal regions of the epithelial cells thus exposing the sensitive rod outer segments to incoming radiation; this is further aided by the contraction of rods in darkness (Fig. 5.2). Cytoskeletal elements (Fig. 5.4) may once again contribute to the migration of the pigment granules.

Pigment migration may, indirectly, have another function in

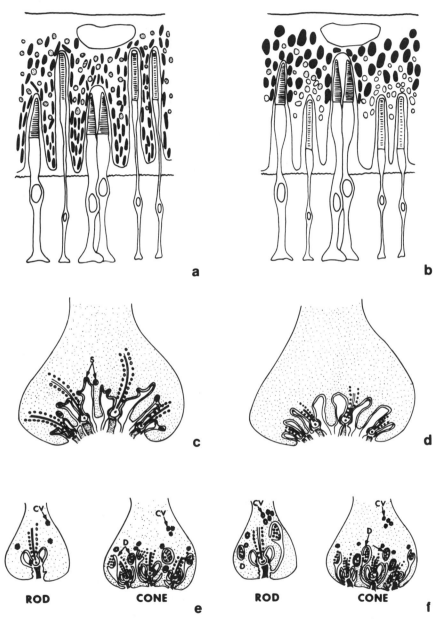

Fig. 5.2: Schematic representation of photomechanical changes in light- (left) and dark- (right) adapted retinas. a, b show positional changes in photoreceptors and pigment granules (■■■). Tapetal spheres (∴∴) in retinas containing a

determining the amount of light striking the photoreceptors. In certain vertebrates (e.g. teleosts), reflecting materials are found within the epithelial cells (retinal tapetum lucidum) (see Chapter 7). In the light-adapted state pigment granules of the RPE migrate between the reflective spheres of the tapetum lucidum, covering their reflecting surfaces and hence screening off reflexions. In darkness, however, when the pigment granules are basally located the reflecting spheres are exposed to incoming radiation (Fig. 5.2). They are thus able to reflect the incident light back over the photoreceptors thereby increasing sensitivity by the additional probability of capture. In elasmobranchs, reflecting material is found in the choroid, and is occlusible (See Chapter 6; Fig. 6.13).

Absorption by Visual Pigment

In order to excite the visual cell, light (photons) has to be absorbed by the visual pigment. Significant bleaching of visual pigment requires quite high light intensities; but is roughly proportional to the number of quanta absorbed. Subsequent regeneration of rod visual pigment is usually complete after about 40 minutes in the human, while cone pigments require about 7 minutes. Thus, in the human, the process of light-adaptation is much faster than that of dark-adaptation. We are fully aware of the disadvantage we are at when we enter a darkened place after being in well-lit surroundings. On the other hand, when the situation is reversed we do not find ourselves at such a disadvantage. This relationship between the amount of photopigment bleached and adaptation was realised since Kühne (1878) showed that the process of dark-adaptation was delayed following exposure to bright light.

---

tapetum lucidum are exposed in the dark. **c, d** show changes in the length of synaptic ribbon and number of spinules (S) (or digitations), coated vesicles (CV) and diverticulae (D). Between 3-5 hours of light adaptation (**e**) maximum number of coated vesicles and diverticulae are present in cone pedicles, the quantity falls off with both shorter and longer periods of light-adaptation; in rod spherules coated vesicles and diverticulae are minimal during the light-adapted state. After 1 hour of dark-adaptation both cone pedicles and rod spherules contain the maximum number of diverticulae and coated vesicles (**f**).
(From Ali & Klyne, 1983)

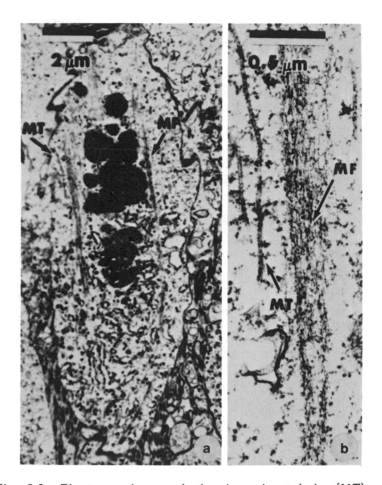

Fig. 5.3: Electron micrograph showing microtubules (MT) and
microfilaments (MF) in a rod photoreceptor of dark-adapted
<u>Salvelinus fontinalis.</u>

The above would imply a link between visual pigment and
adaptation. It has been suggested that adaptation may be initiated
by one or more of the photoproducts of rhodopsin rather than the
visual pigment itself (Donner & Reuter, 1968). However, studies
employing hydroxylamine, to accelerate the photochemical reactions of the isolated retina, showed that it is rhodopsin which is
involved in adaptation (Brin & Ripps, 1977). Furthermore, there is
a logarithmic relationship between receptor sensitivity and concentration of bleached pigment (Fig. 5.5).

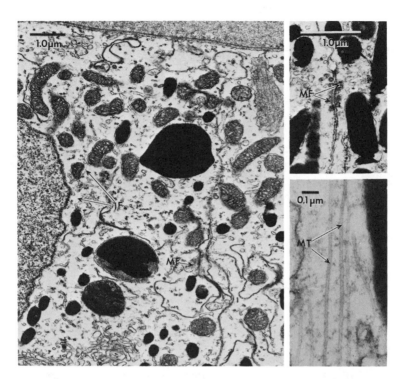

Fig. 5.4:   Electron micrograph showing microtubules (MT), microfilaments (MF) and intermediate filaments (IF or 10-nm filaments) in the retinal pigment epithelium.

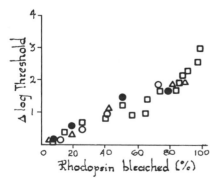

Fig. 5.5: Relationship between the concentration of bleached rhodopsin and the threshold of receptor responses of isolated retinas of axolotl (solid circles), frog (open circles and triangles), and rat (open squares). Note that in the isolated retina pigment regeneration does not occur.
(After Grabowski & Pak, 1975)

For all photoreceptors (vertebrates and invertebrates) there are large components of adaptation which are not correlated with any photometrically measurable changes in visual pigment. Conversely, there may be changes in visual pigment molecules which are not reflected in a change in the absorption spectrum and such changes may be correlated with adaptation.

Neural Processing

There are numerous examples which indicate that higher-order neurones contribute to adaptation. This is related to the difference in neural processing within light- and dark-adapted retinas as illustrated below:-

Light-Adapted	Dark-Adapted
Cones	Rods
Centre-surround	No centre-surround
Fast flicker-fusion	Slow flicker-fusion
Colour vision	No colour vision
Little summation	Much summation

The above illustrates the shift in functioning of the photoreceptors and the subsequent relay of the impulses along different tracks to the brain. This method of retinal adaptation to light and dimness is the least understood, but likely to prove the most important mechanism in light-/dark-adaptation.

Of special interest is the course of human dark-adaptation (Fig. 5.6) which entails integration of information from the two types of photoreceptors - rods and cones. Experimental evidence indicates that, indirectly, the observed kinetics are largely, if not solely, due to the receptors themselves. Following dim-adapting lights that photoactivate only rods, visual threshold recovers in two steps - a fast initial phase ($\simeq$ 1 min) followed by a slower phase ($\simeq$ 20 min). Increasing the adapting intensity leads to cone stimulation and thus to their contribution to dark-adaptation. Since their recovery is much faster than rods, a prominent plateau is observed in the recovery curves (Fig. 5.6). The rods do not contribute because their thresholds exceed those of the cones. With the brightest adapting lights (Fig. 5.6) more than 15 min elapses before

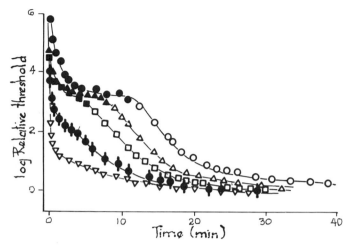

Fig. 5.6:   The course of human dark-adaptation following different degrees of light-adaptation.   Threshold was the intensity of the violet test light that enabled an opaque black cross to be seen.   The log relative adapting intensities were: ●, ○, -3,18; ▲, ▵, - 2,17; ■, ◻, - 1,87; ◆, - 1,16; ▽, - 0,00.   The intensities used were sufficient to bleach from 0,35 to 99,6% of the rhodopsin.   The filled symbols indicate that a violet colour was apparent at threshold, whereas the open symbols indicate that it was colourless.
(After Barlow, 1972)

the rods begin to mediate vision and more than 30 min is required for them to regain their absolute threshold.   This is contrary to cones which recover within 5 to 10 min.

6

ADAPTATIONS TO VARIOUS MODES OF LIFE

The earth's revolution on its axis around the sun results in a 24-hour cycle composed of light (day) and darkness (night) with twilight (dawn and dusk) periods between. The lengths of these periods vary with season and latitude. Within the tropics, especially along the equator, there is practically no variation in the photoperiod (a constant light/dark period of approximately 12 hours each throughout the year) while in the polar regions there can be days in summer that are composed of 24 hours of daylight. Semi-tropical and temperate regions exhibit variations which are intermediate of the two extremes.

Animals, vertebrates in particular, have not only adapted to survive but to succeed under these periods of photic variations. Evolution of adaptations to the various periods is the result of adaptive radiation that lessens competition. For example, an animal that is diurnal (daytime) could become nocturnal (night-time), or vice versa, in order to reduce competition for food or danger from predation. This change in the animal's mode of life is also reflected in its ocular adaptations; indeed so close is this relation that one can predict, with reasonable assurance, something of the habits of the animal as well as its visual ability from the structural organisation of the eye, primarily the retina.

The Diurnal Habit

Most strictly diurnal vertebrates, with the possible exception of snakes, depend more on vision rather than on smell, touch or hearing. Blindfolded birds will fly if released in the air but they cannot alight properly. They cannot orient themselves correctly to the direction and feel of the wind as do normal birds (Beacher, 1952).   Thus, flight of birds is apparently dependent on vision. Strictly diurnal species are functional only during the hours of daylight, with even twilight illumination being unstimulatory. Diurnal birds roost at sunset, and at least one of the ground squirrels does not emerge from its burrow in the morning until the sun's rays are actually over the burrow's mouth, nor can it find its way home if released from a trap in the twilight (Linsdale, 1946). This insensitivity of the eye is reflected in its ocular structure. The diurnal eye works at relatively high illumination, thus acuity (resolving power) rather than sensitivity is of the order.   The first requirement for high acuity is a big image covering as many visual cells as possible, and the first requirement for a big image is a big eye.

Eye: Size and Shape

The diameter of the visual cells does not vary greatly throughout the vertebrates, thus it is the absolute, rather than the relative, size of the eye that matters (Fig. 6.1).   Big animals are likely to have big eyes, but small diurnal animals also tend to have eyes which are relatively large.   This is particularly true of the birds whose eyes are relatively enormous, as big as the head can accommodate.   Diurnal birds' eyes may not look so big on casual inspection because the cornea and lid opening are relatively small, however, upon dissection of such an eye one can see that the posterior chamber is often much enlarged compared with the anterior chamber (Fig. 6.2).   Under such situations the lens is much flattened in order to increase its focal length because the retina is now further from it.   This results in an enlargement of the retinal image at the expense of brightness but this does not matter as the diurnal eye receives plenty of light under its normal working conditions.

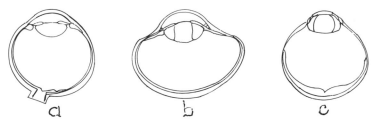

Fig. 6.1: General eye structure of three diurnal species: **a** - monkey; **b** - homing pigeon; **c** - chameleon.
(After Walls, 1942)

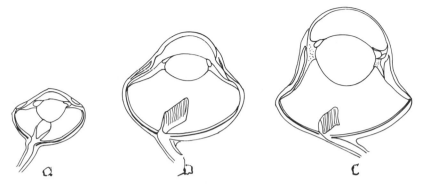

Fig. 6.2:   Birds' eyes showing characteristic shapes. a - commonest 'flat' type (swan, Cygnus olor); b - 'globose' type (eagle, Aguila chrysaëtos); c - 'tubular' type (owl, Bubo bubo) (After Walls, 1942)

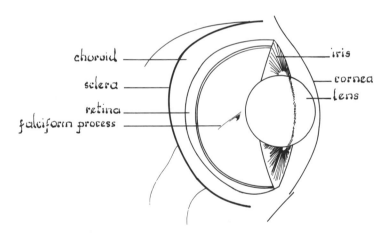

Fig. 6.3:   Diagrammatic view of the eye of a Northern pike (Esox lucius or E. estor) - a diurnal fish.

In diurnal fishes, where the refractive index of the lens is unusually high to compensate for the physiological lack of a cornea, the image formed is broad and so the posterior chamber has not been increased in depth, instead the eye is flattened so that it takes less room in the head (Fig. 6.3).

Pupil

The diurnal eye operates under high illumination, thus the pupil can be relatively small. This is advantageous for visual acuity because it helps reduce the spherical aberration of the less optically perfect lens edges. The pupil of diurnal species is usually circular and shows much less change in size with changes in ambient illumination (Fig. 6.4). Birds have extremely active pupils but, the bird iris is relatively insensitive to light. This has led to the suggestion that the bird's pupil is under voluntary control, birds are unique in that the iris muscles are striated. The bird's (in any case the parrot's) pupil contracts as an interesting object approaches its eye, however, it is not known if this is a reflex contraction linked to accommodation as it is in man. In man, accommodation, pupil contraction and convergence reflexes are linked so that there is always convergence and pupil contraction when the eye accommodates on near objects. Birds, on the other hand, have little eye movement and although some are said to be capable of a slight convergence, there is no convergence on an approaching object in the parrot.

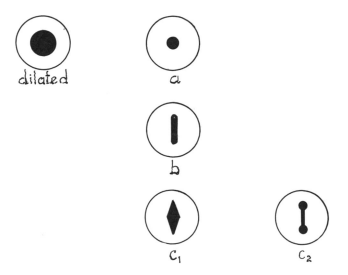

Fig. 6.4:   Round pupil of diurnal and strictly nocturnal mammals.   Contraction may be symmetrical as in man, monkey, dog, arctic fox, jackal, lion, tiger, wolf, owl (a), or asymmetrical, resulting in a vertical slit, as in the British fox and silver fox or the cat (c_1, c_2).

Intra-ocular Filters

All diurnal eyes have some sort of intra-ocular filter, usually yellow, but orange and red filters are also present. These filters take several forms: from the yellow corneas of some diurnal fishes to the coloured droplets in the cones of lizards, turtles and birds.

Cornea and Lens

It has long been known that the corneas and lenses of some vertebrates are yellow in colour and thus they affect the spectral composition of the light reaching the retina (Fig. 6.5). These filters aid in the preferential reduction of light of shorter wavelength from reaching the retina thereby aiding in the reduction of chromatic aberration (less marked at longer wavelengths), scatter (short wavelengths are more easily scattered), and "glare", as well as increasing the contrast of objects viewed against certain backgrounds.

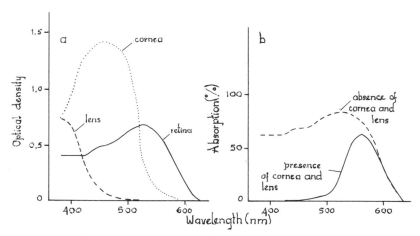

Fig. 6.5: (a) - Spectral absorbance of cornea, lens, and retina of Astronotus ocellatus. (b) - Absorption of incident light by visual pigment alone (absence of yellow cornea and lens) and by the visual pigment in life (i.e. when cornea and lens have the characteristics shown in (a). Note that the position of maximum sensitivity is shifted to about 560 nm. (After Muntz, 1975)

Yellow corneas are particularly common in fishes and are a frequent characteristic of cichlids, wrasses (Labridae), parrot fish (Scaridae), trigger fish (Balistidae) and puffer fish (Tetraodontidae) (see Muntz, 1975). These fishes are highly diurnal and often show specialised methods of passing the night inactive (e.g. wrasse - lying on their sides and burying themselves in sand; parrot fish - remaining immobile after secreting a mucous envelope around themselves). The yellow corneas absorb maximally between 400 nm and 500 nm (Fig. 6.5). The pigmentation is deeper in the dorsal part of the cornea and this is thought to be related to the greater intensity of downwelling as opposed to upwelling light.

Yellow lenses are the oldest form of colour filters known, since they are found in the lampreys. But the possession of a yellow lens does not necessarily mean that the species is primitive because the yellow lens is also a form of secondary development. If other types of intra-ocular filters, particularly coloured oil droplets of photoreceptors, are lost during a period of ancestral nocturnality lens pigmentation is the easiest form of intra-ocular filter development. Yellow lenses are considered a form of secondary development in snakes, some diurnal geckos and some diurnal squirrels. Snakes developed from lizard ancestors and passed through a nocturnal phase during which the eye underwent degeneration, this included the loss of the coloured oil droplets in visual cells. Upon returning to a diurnal habit snakes developed a yellow lens as a substitute for the oil droplets. Diurnal geckos also passed through similar phases. Oil droplets are absent from photoreceptors of nocturnal geckos, while one diurnal gecko (Phelsuma) has only few colourless oil droplets but possesses a yellow lens. The lack of oil droplets and presence of a yellow lens in squirrels suggest that this species also became diurnal second-arily. Yellow lenses are also present in two perciform groups of fishes - wrasses and parrot fish (Muntz 1975), as well as the deep sea fishes Chlorophthalmus spp. (Denton, 1956) and Argyropelecus affinis (see Somiya, 1976). The presence of a yellow lens in man appears accidental but it is nonetheless useful in diurnal vision. Pigmentation of the human lens increases with age and is attributed to the degradation products of proteins (McEwen, 1959).

Generally, yellow lenses and corneas occur together: yellow lenses generally start to absorb at the shorter wavelengths where the corneas start to transmit again (corneal absorption 400 - 500 nm; Fig. 6.5a). Thus, in species possessing both yellow corneas and lenses, wavelengths of shorter than 500 nm will be almost totally prevented from reaching the retina (Fig. 6.5b).

There are two aspects of vision which are probably improved by yellow filters, namely the reduction of contrast through scattering, and the effects of chromatic aberration. On clear days or in clear waters, light scattering follows Rayleigh's law (intensity (i) of scattered light is inversely proportional to the fourth power of the wavelength (λ)).

$$i \propto \lambda^{-4}$$

On hazy or foggy days, or in turbid waters the scattering particles are large and scattering is independent of wavelength, in these cases yellow filters would be less beneficial. The visual range of terresterial objects is greater for long wavelengths under high light intensities (Middleton, 1952). Thus, the presence of yellow filters in the eyes of terresterial vertebrates will improve the visibility of very distant objects on clear days. While this may be important for some diurnal birds it is difficult to believe that the same importance can be attributed to the yellow filters of other terresterial vertebrates. In water, the image forming light from the object is attenuated in its passage through the water by being both absorbed and scattered out of the light beam, while at the same time the water between the object and the observer scatters diffuse veiling light into the eye. Thus, in clear waters, yellow filters increase the contrast of objects against their backgrounds since scattering occurs predominantly at shorter wavelengths.

A second way in which yellow filters may be beneficial is through the reduction of chromatic aberration. Yellow filters substantially reduce the effects of aberration both by shifting the sensitivity to longer wavelengths, where the chromatic aberration is less marked, and by narrowing the spectral range.

Although yellow corneas and/or yellow lenses are the characteristics of diurnal animals, to whom sensitivity is not a problem, yellow lenses have also been found in the benthic deep sea fish, Chlorophthalmus spp. (Denton, 1956), and the mesopelagic deep sea fish, Argyropelecus affinis (Somiya, 1976). Here they serve an ecological function different from that of the yellow lenses of diurnal animals. At these depths solar radiation is practically negligible and bioluminescence or "living light" is more important ecologically. Bioluminescence can be from different regions of the spectrum. Argyropelecus olfersi emits a "yellowish-green" light while the larger predatory stromiatoid emits a red light. Thus, it has been suggested (Somiya, 1976) that the yellow lens of Argyropelecus plays an important role in the detection of longer wavelength light sources (the yellowish-green colours of its own genus and the red light of the predators) against the blue flashes generated in the deep scattering layers.

Oil Droplets

Coloured oil droplets situated at the outer ends of the cone inner segments are a feature of diurnal animals (see Figs. 2.4, 6.6). They are found in the frog, lizards, turtles, birds and marsupials. Oil droplets, when present, in nocturnal animals are colourless. The function of yellow oil droplets is to minimise the effects of chromatic aberration by eliminating the shorter wavelengths of the spectrum.   They also serve to reduce the glare caused by the scattering of short wavelength lights by the atmosphere, hence

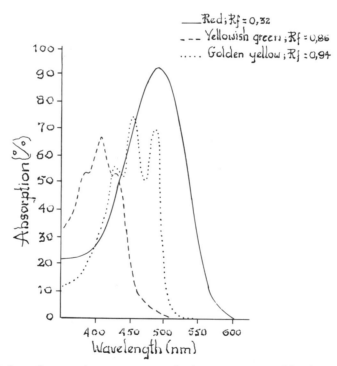

Fig. 6.6:   Apsorption spectra of three carotenoid pigments separated from the chicken retina by thin-layer chromatography (TLC) using benzene as solvent.   Rf values (TLC, chloroform as solvent) for each pigment are also indicated. (After Meyer et al., 1965)

enhancing contrast especially among the green hues which are so prevalent in natural surroundings. Red oil droplets of birds are thought to serve the elimination of Rayleigh scattering which occurs at sunrise and sunset. There is some support for this idea in the fact that early risers among birds (e.g. song birds) have more red droplets than later risers (e.g. hawks) and these again have more than the crepuscular swifts and swallows. This explanation will not account for the red oil droplets of turtles. These animals have, however, to contend with glare over the water and here both their red and yellow filters can be helpful. The kingfisher, which also experiences glare over the water, has a higher percentage of red oil droplets than any bird so far examined (see Chapter 9).

Retina

No other ocular structure is as closely correlated to the mode of life of the animal as is the retina; so much so one can predict with reasonable assurance the habit of the animal from a histological examination of its retina.

The diurnal retina shows a preponderance of cones and sometimes does not contain rods at all (Fig. 6.7). In a comparison of the retinas of birds of different habits it was found that the more diurnal species, in this case the fulmar petrel and the house sparrows, had more cones and less convergence of visual cells on to the ganglion cells than the Manx shearwater, which is unusual among birds in being active by day and night (Lockie, 1952). Pure cone retinas are found in diurnal reptiles and, among mammals, in the diurnal Sciuridae, i.e. the tree and ground squirrels, chipmunks, prairie dogs and marmots; the flying squirrels are nocturnal and are said to have a nearly pure rod retina. The only other strictly diurnal mammals known are the agouchis, South American rodents related to the cavies. These animals are suspected of having colour vision but their retinas have never been examined. Diurnal birds have mixed retinas, with many more cones than rods, but diurnal fishes actually have more rods than cones although here the rods are slender. Except in certain specialised areas which will be considered below, the cones are thicker than the rods and therefore fewer can be accommodated in a given retinal area. This means fewer visual cell nuclei and, in consequence, a thinner outer nuclear layer which may be anything from one (snakes) or two (turtles, squirrels) to several (lizards, birds) cells thick (Fig. 6.7). Because there are fewer visual cells and so fewer synapses to accommodate, the outer fibre layer is also thin in diurnal retinas (Fig. 6.7). Perhaps the most striking thing about the diurnal (and especially the pure cone) retina is the greater thickness of the

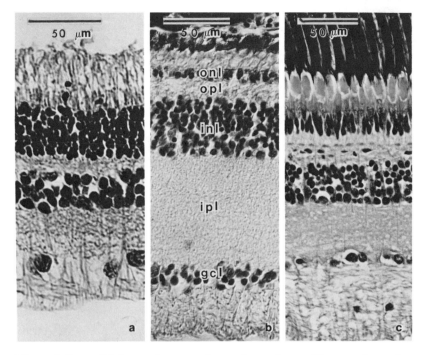

Fig. 6.7:   Light micrographs of retinas illustrating the
adaptations to different habits: **a** - nocturnal (rabbit, no
pigmented epithelium is present as it was an albino); **b** -
diurnal (lizard); **c** - arhythmic (Arctic charr). Note differences
in thickness of the nuclear layers (onl, inl), the synaptic layers
(opl, ipl) and ganglion cell layer (gcl).

inner nuclear layer (Fig. 6.7). Of course, one would expect a good
number of bipolar cells if each visual cell is to have its "private
line" to the optic nerve, but the number of cells in the inner
nuclear layer of a diurnal retina is much more than would satisfy
this requirement.   It is not certain whether there are more bipolar
cells than there are visual cells, but there is certainly a great
increase in the number of horizontal and amacrine cells.   The
function of these "associational" cells is not exactly known, but
they apparently improve the detail of the visual image by
enhancing contrast phenomena.   In a pure cone retina the number
of ganglion cells may equal the number of visual cells, at least in
specialised areas, and the inner and optic nerve fibre layers are
always thick.   In these retinas too the processes of the pigment
epithelium, which extend inwards to the level of the cone ellipsoid,

are full of screening pigment granules so that each outer segment is optically isolated from its neighbours. The pigment granules do not alter their positions in response to changes in the external environment (see Chapter 5).

All diurnal retinas have a specialised area of one shape or another where inner nuclear and ganglion cell layers are thicker than in the rest of the retina. This specialised area is known as the area centralis although it is not always centrally placed. If the retina is a mixed one, as in birds, the rods are absent from this area and the cones may be more slender and longer. Where the cones are thinner, more are packed into a given space and the thickness of the outer nuclear layer is thereby increased. In those retinas which are the most highly developed for visual acuity the area centralis contains a pit or depression known as the fovea centralis. Here the cells of the inner retina are displaced sideways making a deeper or more shallow pit with steeper or more gradual slopes at its edges (Fig. 1.6). In mammals, where the retina is vascularised, blood vessels are excluded from the vicinity of the fovea. It is usually believed that the foveal pit is designed to facilitate the passage of light on to the cones by thinning the retina in front of them, but there have been other theories as to the function of the foveal depression. One theory (Walls, 1937) suggests that the actual shape of the fovea produces a slight magnification of the retinal image owing to the fact that the refractive index of the retina is higher than that of the vitreous (Valentin, 1879a, 1879b). The other (Pumphrey, 1948) points out that a deep fovea will distort an image that does not lie on its centre and that this might serve as a stimulus for correct fixation. Foveas are only present in man and the primates among mammals and even here they are not very highly developed. Some people (Walls, 1940) believe they are degenerate. Foveas occur in such sharp-sighted species as lizards and some teleost fishes but, with the possible exception of lizards, they are most highly developed in birds. Most birds have their eyes placed laterally in the head and their foveas placed centrally in the retina so that their most acute vision will be to the side. However, many birds (hawks, eagles, humming birds, bitterns and various passerine species including swallows) which are especially well-equipped visually, and particularly those which hunt on the wing and need a good distance judgement, have a second fovea (Chievitz, 1889) in a posterior temporal position which can be used in conjunction with the other eye for binocular vision. This lateral fovea is seldom as well developed as the central one. In some birds, both with and without foveas, the area centralis is a ribbon-like formation running across the retina in a roughly horizontal direction. In the lapwing, oyster-catcher, coot, snipe and herring gull it has been shown that, although the position of the bill is very variable between these species, when the head is carried in its normal position during life this special area, as well as the semi-circular canal, is always horizontal (Duijm, 1959). This finding suggests a visual aid to giving the bird a plane of reference in relation to the horizon. Such a ribbon-like central area has never been found in forest inhabitants or birds of prey but occurs mainly in birds of open spaces. It has been suggested that it may be of importance in navigation (Pennycuick, 1960).

An area centralis is very common in teleost fishes and several of these also have a fovea from which double cones are excluded. The teleost fovea is usually laterally placed in the temporal retina and, since fish eyes tend to protrude from the head, this will give its owner foveal binocular vision straight ahead. There is no fovea in any amphibian or, among the reptiles, in crocodiles and alligators or most turtles, although these all have an area centralis which, however, contains rods as well as cones. Diurnal lizards have superb foveas, perhaps as good as those of birds, but most snakes have none. Although mostly diurnal, snakes have poor visual acuity owing to their very small eyes and very big cones. Two snakes only have been positively shown to possess a fovea, the East Indian long-nosed tree snake and the African bird snake. In these the eyes are lateral as in all snakes and the fovea is in the temporal retina. There is a special forward prolongation of the pupil making it keyholed in shape. A line through the fovea and the centre of the lens passes through the pupil prolongation and along a groove in the cheek in front of the eye, thus giving forward binocular vision. It is significant that the East Indian snake is agreed to have the best sight and distance judgement of any snake in the world.

The thinning of the foveal cones enhances visual acuity by packing more visual cells into a given space on the retina (Fig. 1.6). Their increase in length, which especially affects the outer segments, has two further advantages. The retinal image is focussed on to the visual cell outer segments, but the exact position along the length of the outer segment is immaterial. The longer the outer segments the more latitude there is in positioning the image. Therefore, if the outer segments are long, accommodation need not be so precise. For the same reason, long outer segments will diminish the effects of chromatic aberration.

There is no retinal tissue at the site of entry of the optic nerve into the eye, and the nerve-head, therefore, produces a blind spot in the visual field. Where the optic nerve is thin (and this is only in predominantly rod eyes with inferior acuity) the blind spot is unimportant and where the eyes are frontally placed and the visual fields overlap, as in our case, one eye fills in the blind spot of the other. But in diurnal animals the optic nerve is big because of the increased number of ganglion cells and if the eyes are lateral the blind spot could be dangerous. In animals with lateral eyes and big optic nerves this situation is dealt with by flattening the nerve-head into a ribbon and sometimes by moving it out of the way. In diurnal birds and fishes the nerve-head is flattened and in birds it is tucked away under the pecten so that there is only one blind area instead of two. In the diurnal squirrels, the nerve-head is also flattened and, in addition, it is moved into the upper part of the retina, leaving the upper visual field (all images are inverted by the eye's optical system) uninterrupted. It is from the sky that most squirrel species can expect their predators and this arrangement gives them an unimpaired view of it.

The Nocturnal Habit

The nocturnal habit is a form of secondary adaptation. Animals took to the dark to escape competition for food and space, or to find refuge from diurnal predators. Often the predators followed their prey into the night so that although most strictly nocturnal species are those which are preyed upon there are also nocturnal predators. Generally, predators have reasonably good vision, while nocturnal species (especially small mammals) have sacrificed all visual capacities except sensitivity. These animals depend more on smell, hearing and touch than on vision. Mostly they are vegetarians, feeding on foliage and heads of grain. When a species is insectivorous it catches food in bulk as does, for example, the anteater with its sticky tongue. The dependence of strictly nocturnal species on senses other than vision can be observed in certain strains of rats which undergo retinal dystrophy which leave the animals blind soon after the eyes are open in the young. Such animals cannot be distinguished, by observing their behaviour, from their normally sighted companions under daylight conditions in the laboratory. However anyone can recognise a blind kitten from its behaviour.

In addition to the hours of darkness there are other lightless habitats into which some species have retreated for protection. These include the dark depths of the oceans, under the earth, caves and the bottoms of muddy rivers. Inhabitants of these places   also show ocular adaptations (see Chapter 7).

Eye: Size and Shape

The first essential feature for a good nocturnal eye is that it should be an efficient light collector.   A big eye with no further modifications does not satisfy this requirement. What is needed is a big pupil and this entails a big lens if the spherical aberration of the lens periphery is not to become a problem. These changes lead to a proportionate increase in the size of the cornea as well as the anterior chamber. With large anterior chambers, the optical centre of the eye is moved further back. The deeper the optical centre within the eyeball the smaller but brighter the image will be. The nocturnal eye, then, tends to have a large cornea, a large lens which is often nearly spherical, a large pupil and, as a   consequence, a large anterior chamber (Fig. 6.8). In strictly nocturnal species with poor vision the eyes are small, but in the better-sighted nocturnal species the eyes tend to be as big as the head can accommodate and they often develop a tubular shape (Fig. 6.9). This occurs where there is not enough space for the whole eyeball to enlarge and instead the depth of the posterior chamber is increased but not the retinal area. The relatively small retinal area does not matter so much because the bright image, although larger than in a small eye, is relatively small too. Tubular eyes are always enormous (e.g. as in the owl, the bush baby and most deep sea fishes), are frontally placed and are unable to turn in the orbit. To compensate for the lack of eye movement the head usually has a tremendous capacity for rotation; the owl can turn its head at least 270 degrees, but fishes, of course, have to turn their whole body. Nocturnal species with small eyes and poor vision also exhibit little or no eye movement. This is not because there is no room for the eye to turn in the orbit but because with no central area and a spherical lens there is no need for eye movements. With this type

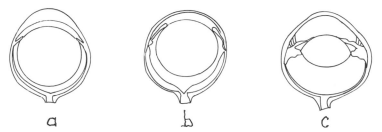

Fig. 6.8: General eye structure of three nocturnal species: a - opossum; b - house-mouse; c - lynx.
(After Walls, 1942)

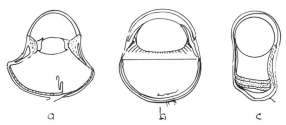

Fig. 6.9: Tubular eyes. Characteristics of nocturnal animals with better vision. An adaptation when there is no room in the head to enlarge the eye further; **a** - owl; **b** - bush baby; **c** - deep-sea fish.
(After Walls, 1942)

of lens, a concentric retina and a large cornea the retinal image is equally good whatever the direction of the external object.

Pupil

A large pupil is characteristic of nocturnal animals. Strictly nocturnal mammals which are content to stay out of bright light have round pupils, being homoiothermic they are relatively independent of the warmth of the sun. Nocturnal animals which emerge during the day and perhaps bask in the sun need more protection from the bright light than that which is afforded by a round pupil. A circular pupil cannot be closed down as far as a slit pupil (Fig. 6.4). In the latter, in addition to the sphincter there are two bundles of muscle fibres which cross above and below the slit and exert a scissors-like action on the pupil, compressing it laterally to the point where it may completely close. Among the mammals only the small cats, some foxes and the doormouse have a vertical slit pupil. Ungulates are not truly nocturnal in habit and generally have pupils in the form of horizontal ovals, which are unable to close completely. In the cat, the edges of the slit meet along most of its length leaving two minute holes one at each end which let in little light but provide pinhole images on the retina. The Chinchilla, which also possesses a vertical slit pupil, shows different degrees of pupil closure under different light intensities. A much more elaborate arrangement occurs in many of the nocturnal geckos. Here the pupil is also round when dilated and a vertical slit when contracted, but there is a series of four notches on each edge of the iris. As these notches are exactly opposite one another four tiny holes are left along the length of the pupil when it is closed. These holes provide pinhole apertures which form a

series of superimposed sharp images on the retina without letting in
too much light.

Most terresterial reptiles like to bask sometimes and those of
them which are nocturnal nearly always have vertically slit pupils;
some very secretive burrowers among the snakes are exceptions.
Amphibians have many bizarre shapes of pupil (Fig. 6.10) but the
truly nocturnal species have slit pupils. Slit pupils may also be seen
in some elasmobranch fishes which like to bask at the surface or in
shallow water. The rays, which often bask, have slit pupils or, in
some species, an operculum (Fig. 6.11). This is a sort of lobe of the
upper iris which can expand and fill the pupil under the action of
light. An analogous structure is often present in whales and also in
the hyrax, while many ungulates have corpora nigra (Fig. 6.11).
These are serrated extensions of the iris, both above and below the

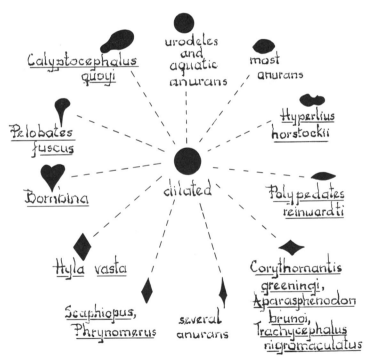

Fig. 6.10: Shapes of the contracted pupil (shown on the
circumference of circle) in different amphibians; all are
circular when dilated (right eyes; not drawn to the same scale).
(After Walls, 1942)

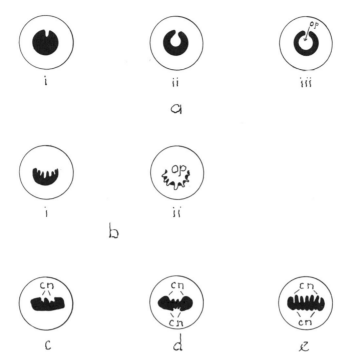

Fig. 6.11: (a) - Various stages (i, ii, iii) in the expansion of the operculum (op) of a loricariid catfish, Plecostomus; (b) - The contracted (i) and expanded (ii) opercula of Raja clavata; (c, d, e) - The horizontal pupils of ungulates and the corpora nigra (cn) along the pupil margins of the horse (c), Gazella dorcas (d) and camel (e).

pupil, which apparently shield the retina from glare either directly from the sky or reflected upwards from the ground. All birds have round pupils whether they are nocturnal or diurnal, the black skimmer, a nocturnal seabird from North America being the only exception.

Retina

The nocturnal retina is always dominated by rods (Fig. 6.7), but only exceptionally, as in the bush baby, the bats, most elasmobranch fishes and the nocturnal snakes and lizards, are there no cones present at all. Nocturnal eyes which are also useful by day (those of the cat and owl for instance) have quite a number of cones, but those of more strictly nocturnal species which normally never emerge after sunrise (e.g. rats, mice and many other small rodents) have so few cones that it is probable that they do not affect vision at all. Such cones as are present are so far apart that they could not provide any reasonable visual acuity even if each had its own connexion to an individual ganglion cell. It is not known whether this does occur in such retinas. Generally, in nocturnal retinas there is an enormous number of long, slender, closely-packed rods showing a great deal of summation on to the bipolar cells, many of which are, in turn, connected to the same ganglion cell. There may be several thousand rods ultimately linked to each optic nerve fibre. Therefore in sections of a nocturnal retina we have a thick outer nuclear layer, an inner nuclear layer which is much thinner, and comparatively few ganglion cells, widely separated, in a single row (Fig. 6.7). The optic nerve fibre layer is, of course, also very thin. The retina is extremely sensitive and the visual acuity very poor. Other retinal modifications for increasing sensitivity can be found in the deep sea fishes. These include banked rods, as found in Bathylagus benedicti and Stomias boa ferox. Banked rods, by increasing the number of photoreceptors within a given area, are thought to enhance sensitivity. Although this may be true it has been shown that in the conger eel, which also possess a banked retina, only the vitread-most layer of the rods function in photoreception while the other layers are thought to act as visual pigment reserves (Shapley & Gordon, 1980). Photoreceptors may also be grouped (e.g. Hiodon) in order to increase sensitivity (see Chapter 7).

We have already seen that nocturnal eyes which are used in daylight usually have a respectable number of cones, but there is one type of pure rod retina which has preserved its visual acuity in another way. In the nocturnal geckos all the cones of their lizard ancestors have been transmuted into rods but in this retina there is much less summation than is usual in nocturnal species. A section through the central retina of one of the nocturnal geckos, Hemidactylus turcicus, shows that the number of visual cells is very nearly the same as the number of ganglion cells. There also appears no summation of rods on to bipolar cells. In addition, the rod synapses of this retina are somewhat complex and more reminescent of the usual cone synapse. It is likely that each rod is connected to more than one bipolar cell. These little lizards have a visual acuity high enough to enable them to catch flying insects by day, but they also become as sensitive as a cat at low illuminations (Dodt & Walther, 1959). This high sensitivity can be partly accounted for by the optical structure of the eye (Tansley, 1959), but it must also be to some extent due to the large amount of visual pigment contained in the massive rod outer segments (Denton, 1956).

Tapetum

The tapetum is a reflecting structure situated sclerad of the visual cells which causes light to pass through the visual cells a second time. The tapetum is responsible for the "eyeshine" of cats, dogs and fishes from turbid waters and the deep seas. As the tapetum is a structure for increasing sensitivity it is never present in a truly diurnal eye.

There are several types of tapetum which may be situated on the inner surface of the choroid or in processes of the cells of the pigment epithelium. In ungulates, some marsupials, elephants and whales the tapetum is made up of tendinous fibres on the inner surface of the choroid. These fibres glisten and reflect the light just like a piece of fresh tendon. In other mammals (e.g. the nocturnal prosimians, the carnivora and seals) the tapetum is still on the inner surface of the choroid but it is cellular - composed of a very regular array of rectangular cells put together like the bricks in a wall (Fig. 6.12). The reflected colours are an interference phenomenon, and the overall effect is usually yellow or green. The bush baby has an extremely vivid yellow eyeshine which is due to a tapetum. The bush baby tapetum is made up of cells packed with pure crystalline riboflavin lying on the inner surface of the choroid. Riboflavin fluoresces blue-green in ultra-violet light and it has been suggested that it enables the bush baby, which has an exceptionally sensitive eye, to utilise the shorter wavelengths, to which it is relative insensitive, by turning them into longer wavelengths nearer the point of maximal absorption of its visual pigment. However, this seems not to be the case for no ultra-violet light reaches the bush baby retina; it is all absorbed in the ocular media. The bush baby tapetum seems just to be an unusually effective mirror. That part of the pigment epithelium which overlies a choroidal tapetum of either type is always devoid of pigment so that there is no interference with the back reflexion of the light.

Some fishes have a fibrous tapetum while others have a special type situated in the processes of the pigment epithelium. This "retinal" tapetum is found in many species inhabiting very turbid waters (e.g. walleye, goldeye; and fishes of the Amazon river and Lake Balaton in Hungary). In the retinal tapetum of teleost fishes the processes of the pigment epithelium cells are packed with crystals of reflecting material which may be classified into

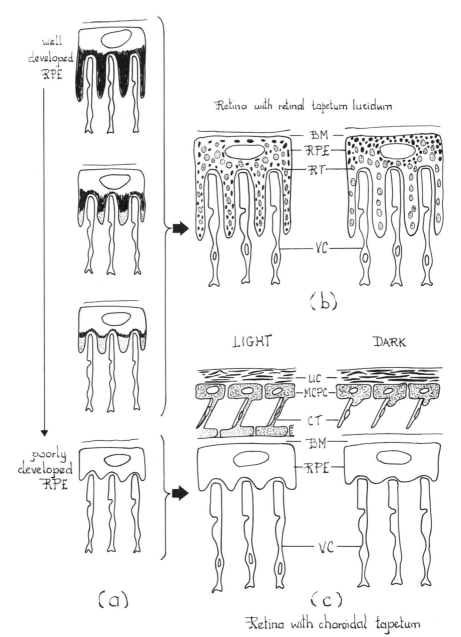

Fig. 6.12: Schematic and hypothetical representation of two processes of tapetal organisation (retinal, choroidal) - retinal tapetum lucida may be found in retinas with well developed

several types depending on their chemical nature; i.e. guanine, uric acid, lipid (glyceryl tridocosahexaenoate), pteridine (7, 8-dihydroxanthopterin) and melanoid (a tetramer of 5, 6-dihydroxyindole-2-carboxylic acid combined with decarboxylated S-adenosylmethionine). This type of tapetum is occlusible in light adaptation, for under these conditions the dark epithelial pigment migrates inwards towards the external limiting membrane, breaking up the reflecting layer and destroying its effectiveness as a mirror (Fig. 6.12; see also Chapter 5, Fig. 5.2). Elasmobranch fishes also have a guanine tapetum, but in these species it is situated in the choroid. It was thought at one time that this tapetum was also occlusible by movements of the choroid pigment, but more recent work (Nicol, 1961) on the dogfish has shown that, at least in this species, there is no movement of choroidal pigment in response to illumination. It was found that the ventral tapetum was permanently occluded while the dorsal tapetum was permanently exposed. It has been suggested that the dark ventral retina which receives light from above has a higher visual acuity, while the dorsal reflecting tapetum increases sensitivity to the much dimmer light coming from below. Choroidal tapeta reported in teleosts appear non-occlusible. The occurrence of non-occlusible choroidal tapeta is apparently restricted to those species inhabiting constantly dim environments. In these species, the choroid lacks the so called "migratory choroidal pigment cells" (Somiya, 1980).

The Arhythmic Habit

Vertebrates are not divided into only two groups - those

RPE, while choroidal tapeta occur in retinas with poorly developed RPE (a). Retinal tapeta may be occlusible (b) and may contain guanine, uric acid, lipid (glyceryl tridocosahexaenoate), pteridine   (7, 8-dihydroxyindole-2-carboxylic acid) or melanoid (a tetramer of 5, 6-dihydroxyindole-2-carboxylic combined with decarboxylated S-adenosylmethionine). Choroidal tapeta, on the other hand, while occlusible in some elasmobranch (c) is non-occlusible in teleosts, in the latter MCPC are also absent.
BM - Bruch's membrane; CT choroidal tapetum; MCPC - migratory choroidal pigmentary cell; RPE - retinal pigment epithelium; RT - retinal tapetum; UC - unmodified part of choroid; VC - visual cell.
(After Somiya, 1980; Walls, 1942)

which are nocturnal in habit. Many species are arhythmic, many
show activity both by day and by night and there are those which
are especially active in the twilight hours around sunrise and
sunset. Arhythmic animals can be found among the teleost fishes,
the frogs, the slit-pupilled reptiles and the larger terresterial
mammals. All these depend on vision (although smell and hearing
may also be important) and have eyes which are adapted to allow
activity under a wide range of illuminations.

The large terresterial mammals, ungulates, elephants and
large carnivores, such as wolves, bears and lions, have no special
retinal or pupillary adaptations such as are found in frogs, teleost
fishes, reptiles and birds. These animals all have mixed rod and
cone retinas (Fig. 6.7). They have large eyes (Fig. 6.13) giving an
extensive retinal area and a large retinal image, but the visual cells
are no bigger than those of small animals. Their rods give them a
good sensitivity at low illuminations, while they have enough cones
to provide a reasonable visual acuity within the large retinal image.
The rather dim retinal image is compensated for by a tapetum
which, in effect, increases its brightness by making it possible to
use the incoming light twice over. Vision is not equally important
to all these species. The elephant, with its relatively small eyes,
can be approached quite close from in front so long as the hunter
makes a minimum of noise and so long as the wind is in the right
direction, while it is important to keep out of sight of a giraffe.
The giraffe eye is, perhaps, the biggest among the vertebrates
although the horse eye runs very close to it. The visual acuity of
the elephant is not nearly as good as that of the horse. For an
elephant to recognise two points as separate they must subtend an
angle of 10 minutes 20 seconds at its eye (Bonaventure, 1961). The
angle for the horse is 3 minutes 15 seconds (Grzimek, 1952) while

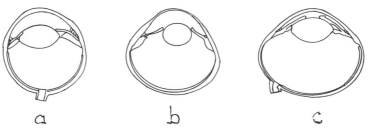

a   b   c

Fig. 6.13: General eye structure of three arhythmic species: **a**
- cougar; **b** - dog; **c** - dromedary.
(After Walls, 1942)

that for the chimpanzee, with its well developed fovea, is only 26 seconds (Spence, 1934). For comparison the relevant angle for the strictly nocturnal rat is 20 minutes (Hermann, 1958). These eyes usually have a central area where the density of the cones is greater and the number of bipolar and ganglion cells is increased. This arrangement reaches its final form in primates and man where a predominantly rod retina, useful for night vision, surrounds a pure-cone fovea with a high visual acuity but a very low sensitivity. The human fovea is virtually night blind while the acuity of the peripheral retina is extremely poor.

Arhythmic vertebrates must be able to react relatively quickly to changes in light intensities. There are two methods by which light reaching the visual cells can be regulated. These are the photomechanical changes (or retinomotor responses) and the changes in pupil size. Generally when one method is well developed the other is usually poorly developed or altogether absent. Pupil changes, when they occur, are usually much faster than the photomechanical reactions and may thus be more useful. In vertebrates where both pupil and retinal movements occur, the faster reaction of the former supplements the more sluggish retinal movements. Phylogenetically photomechanical changes are older and exhibit their highest development in teleost fishes where the pupils are immobile and have no iris muscles at all. As one ascends the evolutionary scale the pupil gradually takes over until in mammals, it has the sole responsibility. Both these methods of regulating light reaching the visual pigments are dealt with in Chapter 5.

Summary

Thus, we see that the vertebrates can be roughly divided into three categories according to their habits with regard to the external illumination level. Firstly, there are the diurnal vertebrates. These have relatively insensitive eyes which are developed for high visual acuity and are incapable of vision at low illuminations. The diurnal eyes tend to be on the large side, to have shallow anterior chambers and deep posterior chambers and to have a retina whose visual cells are predominantly or entirely cones. Diurnal animals always have some type of intra-ocular filters, always yellow but sometimes red and orange as well. These colour filters range from the yellow cornea of really diurnal fishes through the yellow lenses of lamprey, the diurnal geckos, snakes and squirrels to the coloured oil droplets in the cones of frogs, diurnal lizards and birds. In addition, there is the macular pigmentation of man and the primates. Secondly, there are nocturnal vertebrates. These may have large eyes if they are visually oriented (e.g. bush baby, owls) or small ones if vision is relatively unimportant (e.g. rats, mice). The anterior chamber of nocturnal eyes is deep with a large cornea and pupil, and a powerful lens which may even be spherical. The retina is either pure rod or dominated by rods; it also shows much convergence of visual cells on to the optic nerve fibres and is, therefore, very sensitive but visual acuity is poor. The lens and cornea are always colourless and when there are oil droplets in the visual cells these are colourless too. There may be a tapetum. Nocturnal animals, mostly reptiles but also small cats and some fishes and amphibia, which like to emerge in the daylight and perhaps bask in the sun, have extremely active pupils which close, often completely, to a vertical slit. Such a pupil provides excellent protection for a sensitive nocturnal retina. Thirdly, there are vertebrates which are capable of activity at all levels of illumination. In their eyes the proportions of the anterior and posterior chambers are more nearly balanced. The eyes may well be big. The retina always contains both rods and cones, the proportions of these varying with the illumination preferences of the owner. There is usually a specially developed central area in the retina, where the proportion of cones is high, surrounded by a peripheral area of many rods. In man and the primates the central area contains a pure cone fovea. There tends to be some mechanism, photomechanical change or a mobile pupil, for protecting the sensitive rods from being over-exposed to light during the day. There is often a tapetum. There are, of course, all gradations between these three groups. Apart from the nocturnal species with slit pupils there are others which, although night hunters, apparently have good vision during the day. The eagle owl, Bubo bubo, which has been shown to be able to find food by sight in a light too dim to reveal anything to a human observer, can recognise, in full sunlight, diurnal predators invisible to the human eye (Rochon-Duvigneaud, 1943). The little owl, too, can hunt quite successfully in the light although it prefers darkness. Other owls (e.g. tawny owl) seldom appear during the day. Perhaps the eagle owls should be classed as arhythmic animals in spite of their preference for night hunting; they are among the biggest of the owls and have enormous eyes. All owls have a good number of cones although the rods predominate in their retinas. The Manx shearwater is another bird active by both night and day and it is known to possess more rods and to show more convergence in its retina than the strictly diurnal birds (Lockie, 1952). Swifts and swallows also hunt insects on the wing far into the dusk, and must have excellent dim-light vision as well as being perfectly at home in full daylight. Other animals (e.g. rabbits) are mainly active during the morning and evening twilight periods and have no special adaptations for vision at the extremes of high or low illumination.

7

RETINAL ADAPTATIONS TO HABITATS

The organism, a physico-chemical entity, co-exists in delicate balance with its environment. This is manifested not only by external, morphological modifications, but also by structural and physiological changes expressed at tissue and cellular levels. These changes may be divided into two categories:- the first represents a gradual process such as, for example, a unicellular organism evolving into a multicellular one (increase in efficiency); while the second represents a more rapid form of "evolution" whereby an organism adapts to its environment by modifications of pre-existing structures (adaptive radiation). With respect to vision, light (radiation) is the single-most important factor contributing to retinal changes. These changes may, in some instances be rapid enough to be manifested during the life time of the organism, although they may be temporary and revert to the original form once the stimulant is removed.

This chapter will deal with the morphological, physiological and biochemical adaptations of the retinas of vertebrates. Specifically, the emphasis will be placed on functional morphology as it best reflects retinal modifications to adaptive radiation. Although the retinas of all vertebrates will be considered, emphasis will be placed on the retinas of fishes (Super Class Pisces) because they represent nearly half of the living species of vertebrates (about 19 000 out of 40 000). In addition, fishes occupy a wide range of habitats and this diversity is reflected in the retina, of which a much greater variety has been found in fishes than any other class of vertebrates. Retinal modifications will be considered not from a taxonomic aspect, but rather from the point of view of the habitat (Fig. 7.1). In each instance the structure, visual pigment(s) and several established physiological aspects will be considered.

133

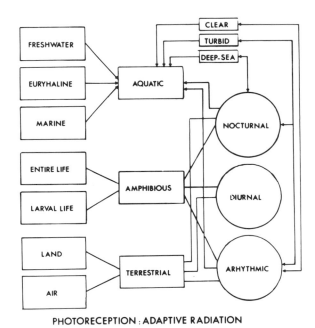

PHOTORECEPTION : ADAPTIVE RADIATION

Fig. 7.1: Diagrammatic representation of the habitats and habits of vertebrates.

Aquatic Medium

This medium may be approached from the salinity and photic aspects. Temperature also influences visual pigments and retinal functions, but it is not an adaptative force in the strictest sense and will be considered only briefly later.

There is a remarkable correlation between visual pigments and the aquatic environment. The rod visual pigment of the freshwater vertebrate is principally porphyropsin (the vitamin A_2 aldehyde (retinal$_2$), 3-dehydroretinal - based photopigment) while in the marine vertebrate it is rhodopsin (the vitamin A_1 aldehyde (retinal$_1$), retinal - based photopigment). Proponents of the theory that vertebrates originated in freshwater state that porphyropsin is the ancestral visual photopigment (Romer & Grove, 1935; Smith, 1932; Wald 1942); while opponents of this theory (Denison, 1956; Crescitelli, 1972) dispute this, and believe that rhodopsin is the ancestral visual pigment since life itself originated in the sea.

Predominance of rhodopsin/porphyropsin is apparent not only in strictly marine/freshwater fishes (Fig. 7.2), but also in migratory fishes (anadromous, catadromous). Catadromous fishes (e.g. killifish, Fundulus heteroclitus; eel, Anguilla spp.) which spawn in the sea, but mature in freshwaters show a predominance of rhodopsin while in the sea and porphyropsin while in freshwater. In contrast, anadromous fishes (e.g. white perch, Morone americana; the sea lamprey, Petromyzon marinus) spawn in freshwater, but spend their juvenile to adult life in the sea. These fishes possess both visual pigments, but exhibit a higher porphyropsin-rhodopsin ratio while in freshwater and the reverse in marine waters.

Although further studies are still necessary, it is apparent that changes in retinal photopigments accompany the metamorphic transitions during the life cycle. Many salmonid fishes perform anadromous migration too, however, the question as to whether or not a phototransition is associated with this migration has not been answered with certainty.

In addition, to the marine-freshwater migration and vice versa, a pigment shift is also manifested in the larval to adult transition of amphibians. Larval amphibians which inhabit a strictly aquatic environment have a porphyropsin rich retina. In some, on maturity, the dorsal (aquatic) retina remains rich in

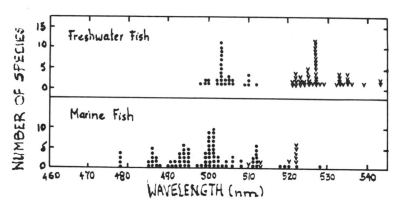

Fig. 7.2: Visual pigment distribution in marine and freshwater fishes. Each point represents the wavelength for maximal absorbance for a single species.
  • -rhodopsin
  v -porphyropsin
(After Crescitelli, 1972)

porphyropsin, while the predominant visual pigment in the ventral (aerial) retina is rhodopsin (e.g. <u>Rana</u> <u>catesbeiana</u>, Fig. 7.3). The four-eyed fish <u>(Anableps anableps)</u> which is also capable of both aerial and aquatic vision (Fig. 4.5) shows not only retinal, but also visual pigment distribution representative of the two media. Rhodopsin is predominant in the ventral (aerial) retina, while porphyropsin is dominant in the dorsal (aquatic) retina.

The electrical activity of photoreceptors in response to incipient light may be recorded from the horizontal cells (S-potential; L (luminosity)-response, wavelength independent; C (chromaticity)- response, wavelength dependent). Comparison of the S-potentials of marine and freshwater fishes shows that in freshwater fishes these responses are shifted towards longer wavelengths (red) while in marine fishes the shift is towards shorter

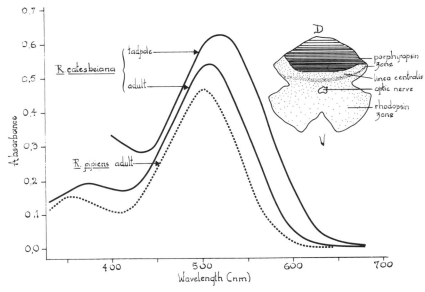

Fig. 7.3: Unbleached retinal extracts from tadpole and adult of <u>Rana</u> <u>catesbeiana</u> (solid curves) and adult of <u>Rana</u> <u>pipiens</u> (dotted curve). The extract of <u>R.</u> <u>pipiens</u> contains only rhodopsin; while the extract of <u>R.</u> <u>catesbeiana</u>, on the other hand, contains almost pure porphyropsin ($\approx 4\%$ rhodopsin). Adult <u>R.</u> <u>catesbeiana</u>, on the other hand, contains both rhodopsin and porphyropsin.
      -see inset for the distribution of these rod visual pigments in the dark-adapted <u>R.</u> <u>catesbeiana</u> retina.
(After Reuter et al., 1971)

wavelengths (blue).   In addition, spectral sensitivity curves, obtained by electroretinography (ERG), may be related to salinity. In general, the maximum peak of these curves is related to the type of rod visual pigment. Thus, in freshwater fishes the peak is at 525 nm or 530 nm, while in marine fishes it is around 500 nm. In migratory fishes òr fishes from estuarine waters the peak is intermediary.   Some workers in this field put forward the hypothesis that the spectral qualities of fresh and marine waters have contributed to the different spectral properties of the retinas of the fishes in these waters.   However, this is not easily explainable, except that oceanic waters show less spectral varia- tion. It is rather more probable that the differences in the spectral properties of the retinas may have resulted from other factors (availability of carotenoids, genetic factors) influencing the choice between the vitamin A_1- and vitamin A_2-based visual pigments.

Photic Qualities

Studies relating retinal adaptations (morphological, biochem- ical and physiological) to photic conditions have proven more fruitful. Organisms inhabiting the aquatic environment are exposed to a wide range of photic conditions, much more so than those in the terresterial environment, and excellent correlations have been established between the functional retinal structure and the environment.

Clear Waters

Light can penetrate to great depths (1 000 metres) in clear waters (Fig. 7.4), however, the spectrum varies with depth (Fig. 7.5) and transparency (Fig. 7.6).

Fishes inhabiting clear, surface waters (e.g. salmon, trout) tend to have large, well-developed eyes with retinas rich in both photoreceptors (rods and cones), and well differentiated inner layers (Fig. 7.7).   The retina is arhythmic, and capable of functioning in a variety of light intensities.   Furthermore, the retina is capable of photomechanical changes - photoreceptors and pigment granules of pigment epithelial cells are capable of reacting to the different light intensities (see Chapter 5).

The absorption spectrum of the scotopic visual pigments of fishes dwelling in clear waters shows a maximum at 500 nm for marine fishes and 525 nm for freshwater fishes; exceptions to this are the anadromous, catadromous and other fishes mentioned in the section above (Aquatic Medium). With decreasing transparency,

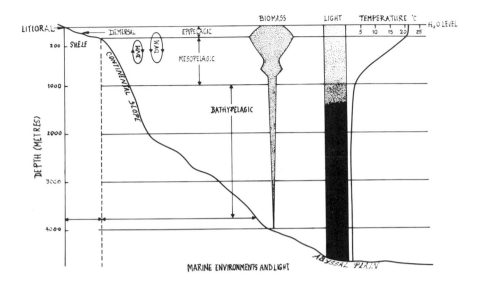

Fig. 7.4: Diagrammatic representation of the relationships between the penetration of light, temperature and biomass at different oceanic depths. The gradient of the ocean bed is exaggerated.
DVM - diurnal vertical migration.
(After Marshall, 1971)

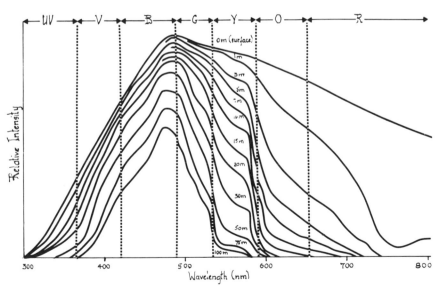

Fig. 7.5: The spectral distribution of solar energy after

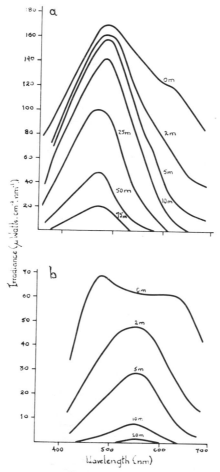

Fig. 7.6: Spectral distribution curves for clear ocean water (east Mediterranean Sea; **a**); peak in blue light ($\approx$ 470 nm) and the ultraviolet is strong even at great depths. An entirely different situation exists in the Northern Baltic Sea **(b)**. The presence of particulate matter and yellow substances shift the maximum transmittance towards 550 nm; ultraviolet is rapidly extinguished in the surface stratum.
(After Jerlov, 1970)

passing through successive depths of distilled water. Note that red and orange radiations are absorbed most strongly while the least affected wavelengths are in the blue.
(After Clarke, 1939)

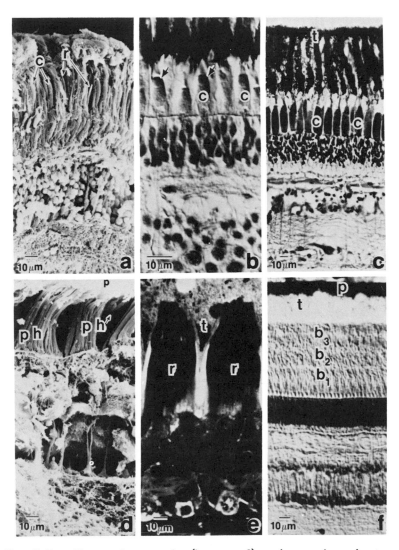

Fig. 7.7.: Photomicrographs (**b, c, e, f**) and scanning electron micrographs (**a, d**) of the retinas of fishes inhabiting different habitats.

a - the duplex retina of the brook trout (<u>Salvelinus</u> <u>fontinalis</u>) which lives in clear waters; **b** - the retina of the killifish (<u>Fundulus</u> <u>heteroclitus</u>) which lives in slightly turbid and green-hued waters, note the oil droplets (arrows); **c** - retina of the walleye (<u>Stizostedion</u> <u>vitreum</u>) which inhabits turbid waters, note the hypertrophic cones and the tapetum lucidum (**t**); **d** -

the absorption maximum of the rod visual pigment, whether it be rhodopsin or porphyropsin, shifts to longer wavelengths. This is true for both marine and freshwater fishes.

A similar distinction is observed in the measurements of spectral sensitivity of marine and freshwater fishes. Flicker fusion frequency (FFF) is much higher in fishes inhabiting clear waters than those in turbid waters. An excellent correlation was established between maximum FFF, the latency and components of the ERG, and the habitat and mode of life of fishes (Fig. 7.8). It is apparent that well-developed inner cellular layers and FFF are influenced by habitat. In other words, the more developed the inner cellular layers, the higher the maximum FFF; and this denotes active fishes living in clear waters. Furthermore, the well-developed inner layers, in relation to the great number of slender cones, suggest that acuity of these animals is high. Thus, the interrelation of cones and horizontal cells may also indicate the habitat and mode of life of fishes.

Turbid Waters

Turbidity of water and air is of different degrees and types. Fig. 7.9) shows the transmission curves (at a 1 metre depth) in oceanic and coastal waters due to turbidity. From the curves it is evident that oceanic waters show less variation than coastal waters. The latter being more under the influence of the type of bed (silt, sand, mud, etc.), turbulence caused by tides, strong currents and surfs, particularly when blown by strong winds. The same range of turbidity may also be found in freshwaters. These waters may be crystal clear (e.g. Lake Malawi in Africa, Crater

---

duplex retina of the mooneye (Hiodon tergisus) which also inhabits turbid waters has grouped photoreceptors (ph) (bundles containing both rods and cones) and a tapetum; e - retina of Scopelarchus guentheri which is a deep sea fish in which the rods of the pure rod retina are grouped into bundles which then act as macroreceptors; f - the pure rod retina of Argentina silus, another deep sea fish, here the rods are slender and are arranged into banks (b_1, b_2, b_3), the pigment epithelium does not exhibit retinomotor movements and the tapetum (t) is well developed.
c - cones;   r - rods;   ph - photoreceptors;   p - pigment;   t - tapetum.
(From Ali, 1981)

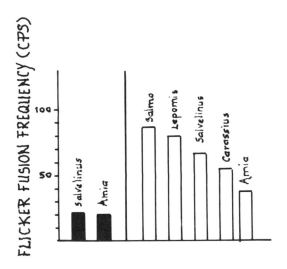

Fig. 7.8: The maximum flicker fusion frequency of the ERG of various fishes in light and darkness. The results were obtained from the same laboratory using similar techniques. Solid bars represent results from dark-adapted samples, and the clear bars from light-adapted samples.
(After Gramoni & Ali, 1970)

Lake in California) on the one hand, or extremely turbid (e.g. Solimôes River in South America) on the other. Between these two extremes a gradient of turbidity may be found. In addition, the waters may also be tinted, for example, by algae, dissolved materials, organic materials in suspension; while red-hued waters is usually the result of the proliferation of plankton or bacteria. Furthermore, freshwaters may show a range of pH (from acid to basic).

Studies on the retinal adaptations of fishes living in turbid waters have been approached from the point of the visual pigments, retinal structure and physiology. Retinas of fishes in turbid waters (Fig. 7.7) usually contain a high number of slender rods and few cones, the latter may be enlarged and contain inclusions (e.g. walleye, Stizostedion spp.) or they may be grouped (e.g. goldeye, Hiodon spp.). In the Hiodontidae, the rods are also grouped with the cones. Droplets or inclusions, the result of hypertrophy of mitochondria, are also observed in the killifish (Fundulus) which inhabits green-hued waters. Further retinal adaptations include the presence of reflecting material in the pigment epithelial cells

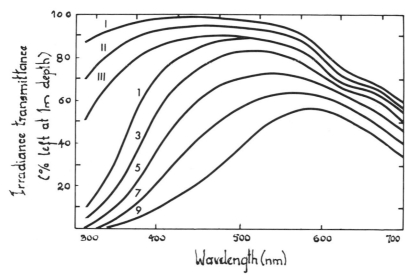

Fig. 7.9: Spectral transmittance of the three basic oceanic water types (I, II, III) and five coastal types (1, 3, 5, 7, 9) for high solar altitudes (areas off Scandinavia and northwestern USA). Note that for the two groups of curves the decrease in transmittance from one type to the next (with increasing numerical value) is most marked in short wave light. This results in a shift from a maximum transmittance from blue, in the clearest waters, over green to brown in the most turbid waters.
(After Jerlov, 1970)

(tapetum). These modifications of retinal structure are thought to be means of increasing visual sensitivity by;- increasing the number of scotopic photoreceptors (rods); converging the incipient light; and increasing the possibility of photon capture by redirecting light entering the retina twice over the outer segments of the photoreceptors. The walleye and goldeye clearly illustrate two morphological modifications employed to solve the same problem (convergent evolution).

An interesting correlation has also been established between visual pigments (rods and cones) and photic conditions. In general, the maxima of the absorption spectra of scotopic visual pigments correspond to the maxima of the transmission spectrum of the water. Thus, the more turbid the water the greater is the shift of the absorption spectrum of the scotopic visual pigment to longer wavelengths (Fig. 7.10).   This is clearly illustrated in the comparative study conducted by Pothier and Ali (1978) on three percids. With respect to the photopic visual pigments (cones), most turbid water fishes lack blue cones which to all intent and purposes are practically useless if the cornea or crystalline lens is yellow. There is another interesting point, the cichlid (Nannacara anomala) which inhabits partially turbid waters lacks green cones, but the rods are large and function both in scotopic and photopic vision as evident from the display of the synaptic ribbons (Ali et al., 1978).

At the physiological level, the ERGs latency (waves **a**, **b**, and **d**) are longer, and the FFF of the ERGs lower in fishes of turbid waters. It is also interesting to note that in fishes such as the walleye (Stizostedion) the maximum FFF is attained at light

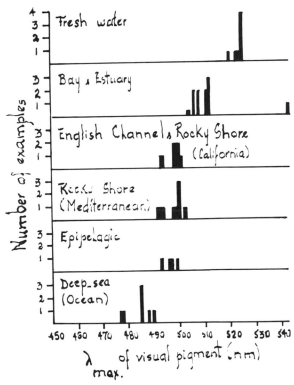

Fig. 7.10: The $\lambda_{max.}$ of visual pigments extracted from eyes of fishes caught in various types of natural waters. (After Lythgoe, 1972)

intensities lower than the threshold intensities necessary to induce the dark-adapted state in the retina of fishes which possess the reflecting material (retinal tapetum) (Ali & Anctil, 1977). From this it is apparent that eyes with reflecting material utilise to the fullest the available downwelling light. In the light-adapted state, on the other hand, the reflecting material is shrouded by the melanin pigments of the retinal epithelial cells and thus there is no difference in the FFF or its maximum of light-adapted fishes containing or not containing reflecting material.

The S-potential of turbid water fishes is also different from that of clear water fishes. The peak of the L-potential is displaced to the red region, while the C-potential, which is bimodal, changes such that the sensitivity in the red is less than the sensitivity in the blue.

Deep Sea

Even in very clear waters light does not penetrate more than 1 000 metres (Figs. 7.4, 7.6). Fishes in these waters may show not only a reduction in the function of the eye, but also in the size of the eye itself. On the other hand, the eye may be enlarged to permit structural modifications of optical structures such as the crystalline lens and cornea (see Fig. 6.9c) as well as the retina (Fig. 7.7f). Measurements of the attenuation of light as one descends show that after a depth of 500 metres only the blue-green light remains. In deeper waters there is barely any light (Fig. 7.4), and vision at these depths is tuned to bioluminescence (inter- and intra-specific). Under these light conditions retinal sensitivity is the key. Thus, cones are superfluous as photopic vision is practically non-existent; instead, rods are modified to augment sensitivity (Fig. 7.7f). The number of rods is increased, these rods are usually slender and arranged in banks; or the rods may have exceptionally long outer segments. These modifications are thought to increase the probability of photon capture by increasing the amount of scotopic visual pigment. In these fishes, photoreceptors may occupy up to 90% of the volume of the retina. Recently, however, a study on the conger eel, which has a banked retina, showed that only the vitread-most layer of rods function in photoreception while the rest were suggested to function as visual pigment reserves (Shapley & Gordon, 1980). No tangible proof was forwarded to substantiate the latter claim. In other instances, the rods may be grouped as in the Hiodon. In this fish the cones are also grouped within the rod bundles (Wagner & Ali, 1978). The inner neural layers of the retina of these fishes are not as well developed, thus reflecting the importance accorded to summation (high sensitivity).

Scotopic visual pigments of fishes inhabiting deep waters are more sensitive to blue light, with the maximum around 480 nm. The maximum absorption spectra of almost all species of deep sea fishes studied do not surpass 500 nm. Although the spectral quality of light reaching a fish has an influence on the spectral character- istics of visual pigments it is possible to find fishes in which the visual pigments differ from the qualities of the ambient light. Nevertheless, these fishes are still well adapted according to the sensitivity hypothesis. Certain fishes (e.g. Pachystomias, a pelagic fish (Denton et al., 1970); Aristostomias scintillans (O'Day & Fernandez, 1974) a bioluminescent deep sea fish) which have photophores emitting red light also have red sensitive photo- pigments in the retina (See also Somiya, 1979).

The physiological studies of the retina of deep sea fishes present certain technical difficulties arising from their capture and maintenance in captivity under conditions representative of the deep sea environment.   Furthermore, these fishes tend to be bloated when brought to the surface because of the rapid reduction in pressure which causes an enlargement (and even bursting) of the swim bladder.

Tide Pools

There appears to be only one documented account of vision in tide pool fishes (Wagner et al., 1976). Ten species from as many families were studied.   They may be classified as permanent dwellers and temporary dwellers. The latter group is composed of juvenile which profit from the protection afforded by this envi- ronment. However, when they mature they abandon this habitat. The typical inhabitants of tide pools may either be active forms which fully exploit their visual capacities, or bottom living forms, or hiding forms.

Based on the observations of the retinal structure of the ten fishes it is apparent that their retinal adaptations may be divided into three broad categories:- (i) fishes dependent on vision (good acuity and sensitivity); (ii) fishes specialised for vision in murky waters or dim light environment (poor acuity and/or high sensi- tivity); and (iii) fishes with poor visual capacity (very reduced acuity and sensitivity).   In the first group the retinas are characterised by regular cone mosaics, high receptor densities and a low degree of summation. At the other extreme, in the third group, the retinal pigment epithelium is sparse, receptor density

low, summation high and integration rates low. Due to the
intermediate nature of the second group, the retinal adaptations
are heterogenous. The common features are low cone densities,
high rates of summation and high degrees of integration. These
may be coupled to specialised features; for example, Labrisomus
nuchipinnis has a reduced retinal pigment epithelium, a well-
developed reflecting layer, conspicuous oil-droplets and prominent
grouped rods (Wagner et al., 1976). Although these features are
present in the other members of the group, they are less
pronounced.

Marshes

Marshes are excellent nurseries for fishes. Evidently the
presence of young fishes would attract predators, however the
young predominate. Most of the species of fishes occupying this
habitat abandon it when mature, but there are also those which
spend their entire lives in the marshes. In general, the waters of
marshes are dimly lit due to the abundance of vegetation, in
addition the water may also be turbid. Thus, the retinal
adaptations of fishes in marshes resemble closely that of fishes
found in turbid and murky waters (Menezes et al., 1981).

Terresterial Environment

Retinal adaptations in terresterial vertebrates (including
aerial and burrowing vertebrates) are related to their habits rather
than their habitats (adaptations to habits were considered in
Chapter 6). It is interesting to note, in passing, the remarkable
similarities between the retinal structure of terresterial vertebrates which occupy different habitats but observe the same habits.
For example, nocturnal animals of different habitats (such as the
mouse, bat and owl) have remarkably similar retinal structure;
rather, ocular adaptations are of the essence. The uniformity of
retinal composition of terresterial vertebrates also extends to the
visual pigments. Spectral distribution of the sun's energy shows a
broad maximum centred at 500 nm (Fig. 5.1) and it is not surprising
that the majority of terresterial vertebrates possess pigments with
λ_{max} within the 493 nm to 502 nm range. The reason for this is
that except under dense foliage, radiation reaching the earth's
surface is modified only by atmospheric absorption. Although this
may vary somewhat from location to location it has a negligible
effect on the spectral energy distribution, therefore negating the
need for variation in visual pigments. The strictly terresterial
vertebrates will be considered here. They will be grouped into the

predator group and into burrowing and aerial animals.

Birds will be taken to represent the predator group. Almost all predator birds (except the owl) are diurnal in their habits. Four striking retinal adaptations observed in diurnal birds are:- (i) the presence of oil-droplets in the cones (these are thought to function as filters, enhancing acuity and reducing aberration); (ii) the ability of both the cones and the retinal pigment to exhibit photo-mechanical responses, the latter method of responding to light of different intensities is usually attributed to the lower vertebrates, however birds have maintained this capacity although they also exhibit pupillary changes (iris response); (iii) the presence of two foveas in birds of prey (e.g. falcon), one for binocular vision and the other for monocular vision, the foveas are also thought to enhance visual acuity; and (iv) the FFF in these birds is also very high.

The eye of burrowing animals is generally small, and the retina resembles that of nocturnal vertebrates - the majority of the photoreceptors are rods; the pigment epithelium is reduced or without pigment granules; and photomechanical movements of the photoreceptors are absent. In other words, it is a retina specialised for vision at low light intensities (high sensitivity).

The third group is composed of tree dwellers such as lizards, squirrels and monkeys; birds too may be included within this group. In this group of vertebrates the retina is adapted for high acuity - high density of cones, low degree of summation, presence of a fovea, and colour vision. Note, however, that colour vision is not limited to this group; birds of prey, fishes, etc., also possess colour vision. Some of the tree dwellers (e.g. monkey) are arhythmic in the sense that they can see in varying light intensities - both at dawn and at dusk. These vertebrates have duplex retinas, rich in both scotopic (rod) and photopic (cone) photoreceptors. These characteristics and aptitudes are carried over to the anthropoids, some of whom are no longer tree dwellers.

Temperature

Temperature is not a factor affecting photoreception in the strictest sense; except that like all other processes (whether they may be morphological, chemical or physiological), there is an upper and lower limit between which the process can occur. Thus, the vision of poikilotherms will come more under the influence of temperature than that of homeotherms. In the foregoing habitats discussed temperature may differ within the habitats. For example, turbid waters may be both cold (temperate regions) or warm (tropical regions); the same holds true for clear waters and terresterial habitats. The only habitat where there is little variation in temperature is within great oceanic depths.

Generally, in a colder environment (particularly true for poikilotherms) the primary visual process is slowed down. Consequently, the threshold is increased; while acuity and the ability to perceive movement is reduced (see Ali, 1975, for review). Furthermore, temperature has been reported to modify spectral sensitivity (Tsin & Beatty, 1977). Changes in the amount of visual pigments as well as the proportion of photopigments in species with paired photopigments are also affected by temperature. In the latter, higher temperature increases the proportion of rhodopsin, whereas lower temperature builds up the proportion of porphyropsin (see Allen et al., 1982; Tsin & Beatty, 1977). The changes in visual pigment levels is associated with the change in rod dimension (e.g. length). The increase in visual pigment levels during winter has been demonstrated in some species (e.g. trout, shiner), and it has been suggested that this leads to greater sensitivity during the dawn and dusk periods; while the increase in the ratio of porphyropsin to rhodopsin leads to sensitivity in the longer wavelengths (Allen et al., 1982). In support of this, changes in visual pigments have been correlated with appropriate changes in visual threshold in the amphibian Xenopus and albino rat (see Allen et al ., 1982).

Temperature was also found to affect photomechanical or retinomotor responses, however, this was evident only in darkadapted animals. At both ends of the temperature scale (0 - 14°C, 19 - 33°C), for frog, pigment granules of the retinal pigment epithelium migrated into the apical processes (i.e. appeared as in the light-adapted state) whereas between 14 - 18°C there was minimal expansion (i.e. as in the normal dark-adapted state). Cones too contracted in darkness at temperatures between 30 - 36°C while 3°C and 16°C had no effect. Rods appeared, relatively, unaffected (see Ali, 1975). The rate of adaptation is also affected by temperature; rate of dark-adaptation for cones and retinal pigment epithelium being extremely slow at low temperatures. Temperature, however, is not a permanent factor affecting retinal structure, rather, photic conditions is one of the chief determining factors.

Summary

In summary, it can be said that there is an excellent correlation between the aquatic habitats and the structure and function of the retinas of fishes; and that retinal structure of terresterial vertebrates is more uniform and reflects their habits rather than their habitats.

It is, however, important to note that other biological parameters besides the habitats must be considered when studying retinal structure and vision. More detailed studies are required to better understand retinal adaptations to the various habitats. These include:- synaptic relations, visual pigments, visual acuity, and the effect of coloured (generally yellow) cornea, oil-droplets and crystalline lens related to the functions of the retina under normal conditions or at threshold light intensities.

8

ACUITY AND SENSITIVITY

All visual information passes through the retina, and the retina then communicates with higher centres of the brain through the optic nerve which consists of individual nerve fibres, each serving a different area of the visual field. Since the individual fibres of the optic nerve cannot accurately signal levels of activity over a range of more than one hundred to one, the retina must compress the very large range of intensities presented by the external world into a narrow range that can be adequately handled by the optic nerve fibres.

In all vertebrates the retina is constructed with the same five basic types of cells (photoreceptors, horizontals, bipolars, amacrines, ganglion cells - Figs. 1.5, 2.1). Information is carried in two directions through the retina. In the input-output direction it is carried in sequence by receptor cells to bipolar cells and on to ganglion cells (Fig. 8.1). The receptor cells which contain the photopigments act as transducers. They convert light energy into nerve impulses which are in turn processed by succeeding cells. Receptor cells drive the bipolar cells which then pass the signal to the ganglion cells. The ganglion cells generate the retinal output; their outgoing fibres comprise the optic nerve which carries the information to the brain. Visual information can also be sent back to the level of the photoreceptors via the biplexiform cells. Information is also spread out laterally, perpendicular to the input-output pathway, by the horizontal and amacrine cells (Fig. 8.1). Each neurone communicates with another at a synapse or junction by releasing a transmitter across the small space between the membranes of the two cells. The transmitter is then stored and later released by synaptic vesicles. A good indication of the site and direction of synaptic transmission is therefore the presence of

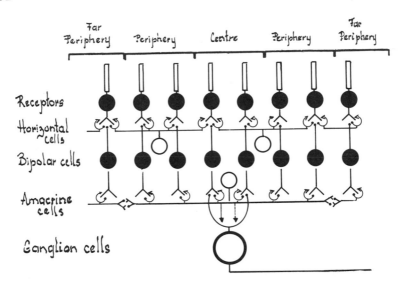

Fig. 8.1:   The "wiring diagram" of a retinal ganglion cell
showing how it is influenced by four cell types, some of which
interact laterally.
➤— -excitatory synapse
→ -inhibitory synapse
(From Dowling & Boycott, 1966)

vesicles within the membrane enclosures of the transmitting cell.
The general scheme of the retinal wiring diagram obtained from
electron microscopic observations is as follows:-   each neurone
receives a message from the cell that precedes it in the input-
output pathway; it in turn is capable of transmitting back to that
cell, across to its neighbours, or forward to the succeeding input-
output cell (Fig. 8.1).   This means horizontal cells can transmit
back to receptor cells, laterally to other horizontal cells, and
forward to bipolar cells.   Similarly, amacrines can transmit to
bipolar cells, other amacrine cells and to ganglion cells. The
functional result of these anatomical relations is that each input-
output pathway is strongly influenced by activity in neighbouring
pathways through the laterally oriented interneurones (Fig. 8.1).
This interplay of the neurones determines to a large degree the
visual capabilities (acuity and sensitivity) of the vertebrate.

Acuity

The resolution of an eye ultimately depends upon the wavelength of the light, and the best resolution of a small eye cannot match the best resolution of a large one. By convention, visual acuity is defined as the reciprocal of the minimum resolvable angle expressed in minutes of arc. In vertebrates visual acuity or resolving power (ability to distinguish fine detail) is a function of the optical quality of the image given by the ocular system, on the one hand, and the anatomical and physiological capabilities of the retina in analysing the image on the other. The quality of the image is governed by diffraction effects at the entrance aperture; while the slenderness, density, and particularly the number of visual cells connected to each optic nerve fibre determine the detail of the image that can be analysed. The human retina, for example, contains approximately $7x10^6$ cones and $120x10^6$ rods; but there are not even $1x10^6$ fibres in the optic nerve to conduct the information received by the photoreceptors to the brain. Although finer retinal grain can be achieved by smaller visual cells, these cells cannot be reduced indefinitely. Photoreceptor outer segments with diameter less than 1-2 μm will cause the light to be guided down the exterior to the cell. Consequently less light is absorbed by the visual pigment molecules and light passing along one visual cell may be absorbed by its neighbour. Thus the two cells cannot act independently of each other. The 1-2 μm value is set by the refractive index difference between the visual cell and its surrounding medium, and by the wavelength of light (see Lythgoe, 1979).

If the images of two point sources of light fall on two visual cells which are sufficiently far apart (i.e. relatively unstimulated cell(s) between them) two different nerve fibres will be stimulated and the point sources will be recognised as separate. The thinner and nearer together these two cells are the closer can the light sources be and still be appreciated as separate. However, when the light sources are close enough such that their images stimulate two adjacent cells, it is impossible to tell that there are two sources rather than one which is large enough to cover both cells. The above argument would not hold if these visual cells were connected to the same optic nerve fibre. In the case of cones, under high light intensities, this does not seem to occur although there are many cross-connexions in a cone retina. In spite of the elaboration of the inner nuclear layer, and the fact that many of the inner nuclear cells appear to be connected to each cone by way of their complex synapses there does appear to be a straight connexion of each cone to an individual ganglion cell and thus to an individual optic nerve fibre.

Visual acuity increases with increase in light intensity, not because the pupil contracts, but, because the central parts of the retina are used. Peripheral areas of the retina contain a higher rod:cone ratio and are more sensitive to light and less accurate as far as acuity is concerned. The central areas of the retina, on the other hand, contain a higher proportion of cones and are thus less sensitive, but, more accurate; the foveal region contains purely cones which are characteristically more slender than cones in other regions of the retina (Fig. 1.6). Areas of retinas with particularly high acuity are found in almost all vertebrates but particularly in mammals and birds (Walls, 1942; Rochon-Duvigneaud, 1943). However, in one and the same region of the retina, visual acuity also varies within wide limits with changes in intensity. Hecht (1928) attributed the increase in visual acuity with increasing retinal illumination to the different sensitivities of individual retinal light detectors. Thus, more detectors are stimulated by light at higher than at lower illuminations. Hecht's original theory was rejected primarily on grounds that it assumed a very wide distribution of light sensitivities among the rods and among the cones. Nevertheless, the general idea that a retinal mosaic can become functionally finer at higher illuminations need not be abandoned.

In humans, the highest acuity value was obtained from a grating (made of equally wide black and white bars) of 2,1 μm which represents a retinal separation of 2,3 μm. The interference fringe technique (dark and light fringes produced inside the eye by the interference of two coherent beams of light), on the other hand, gave retinal acuity values of 2 μm or slightly more than 2 μm for man. While anatomical measurements gave values of 2,0 - 2,5 m for the inter-centre distance of central foveal cones. Despite uncertainty inherent to such comparisons this agreement is strong evidence that for the grating it is the fineness of the cone mosaic which sets the ultimate limit to the acuity of the eye. Humans have been the favourite subjects for the study of visual acuity because they can readily and reliably indicate their visual experience. Psychophysics is a subfield of psychology that quantitatively correlates the physical properties of a stimulus with the evoked human response. Landolt's C (a black letter C against a white background; Fig. 8.2) has been used in psychophysical experiments on visual acuity. Subjects could freely move their heads so that the image of the object viewed falls on the most sensitive retinal regions. At any given background intensity, the letter's dimension was altered until the gap was just resolved (i.e. viewed as C instead of O). The angle subtended by the gap in the

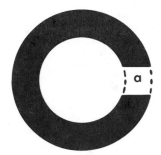

Fig. 8.2: Landolt's C. A black, broken ring of gap **a** against a white background.

letter (**a** in Fig. 8.2) was then the minimum resolvable angle expressed in minutes of arc. Increase in intensity of the white background allowed the experimental subjects to use the foveal region of their retinas. Foveal acuity eventually achieved an angular resolution of 30 sec of arc - an angle subtended by a 0,15 mm large object held at arm's length (Fig. 8.3). This may also be predicted from foveal cone density using the equation below:-

$$\text{Inter-receptor angle} = 2 \tan^{-1} (d/2f)$$
where
  f = focal length of the eye
  d = inter-receptor distance.

Thus, visual acuity of the discernment is apparently the property of cones.

The highest recorded visual acuities of vertebrates belong to the birds of prey; the resolving power of the eagle being two to three times greater than that of man (Shlaer, 1972; see also Chapter 6).

Sensitivity

The other property determined by retinal architecture is visual sensitivity (the ability to detect small quantities of light). In this case, everything is done to increase sensitivity and generally this leads to a loss of acuity.

Studies on absolute sensitivity of the goldfish showed that the rods and red cones of this animal are equally sensitive to light of

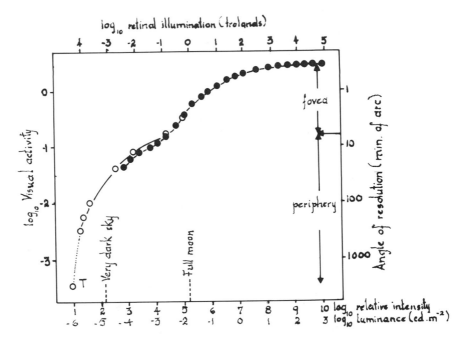

Fig. 8.3: Visual acuity of the freely moving human eye as a function of light intensity, using Landolt's **C** as a visual target. Visual acuity is plotted on the left and the corresponding minimum resolvable angle gives the field illuminance both as relative intensity and candelas per metre square. The upper scale gives retinal illumination in special units, photopic trolands. The break in the curve represents the transition from scotopic to photopic vision. Points marked "very dark sky" and "full moon" refer to the illuminance of the sky under these conditions. Point T corresponds to the absolute threshold luminance for a large field 47° diameter. (After Pirenne, 1967; Fein & Szuts, 1982)

the wavelength 636 nm (Powers & Easter, 1978). However, if the retinal illumination necessary for vision is considered then the rods are about five times as sensitive as the red cones. This may be due to the larger retinal surface occupied by the rods over the red cones; or the higher intrinsic photosensitivity (i.e. voltage/-quantum) and greater inter-receptor connectivity of rods. Sensitivity thus appears to be a property of rods.

If the degree of photon capture and length of outer segment are the same, it follows that a visual cell with an outer segment with a large cross-sectional area will capture more photons and hence be more sensitive than one with a smaller cross-section. Nevertheless a single photon is potentially capable of triggering a response in vertebrate rods (see Miller, 1981). Visual sensitivity may also be influenced by the neuronal circuitry of the retina. The responses of a group of cells may be summed together - in man as many as 300 rods may contribute to one pool (Pirenne, 1967). When summation of this kind occurs, the retina is functionally divided into fewer individual areas, with each area having higher sensitivity. Neural summation is apparently less well developed among cones (Walls, 1942), but as summation increases sensitivity at the expense of acuity this is not surprising. However, it is currently thought that crepuscular predator fishes have adapted for the low light intensities at dawn and dusk by possessing cones with enlarged cross-sectional area outer segments (Munz & McFarland, 1977). Instead of increasing cross-sectional area, sensitivity may also be increased by increasing the density of photoreceptors per unit area. Thus highly sensitive rod retinas may be characterised by a vast number of slender, closely packed rods, or rods arranged into banks (Fig. 7.7). This increase in the number of rods does not contribute to acuity because several of them are connected to each optic nerve fibre. Another adaptation which may be connected with summation is shown by some deep-sea fishes which possess in some areas of the retina tight bundles of rods which are optically isolated from neighbouring bundles by screening pigments e.g. Scopelarchus guentheri, S. sagax (Locket, 1971), and Scopelosaurus lepidus, Evermanalla indica, Ahliesarus berryi (Munk, 1971).

Further modifications for increasing visual sensitivity include pupil size and the presence of a tapetum. Eyes with large pupils are much more sensitive to point sources of light than eyes with small pupils. In the case of a diffused light source, the brightness of the image is related to the diameter of the lens aperture (pupil) and the focal length of the lens:-

$$dq \propto A^2/f^2$$

where
  dq = brightness of a small area of the image
  A   = diameter of the pupil aperture
  f   = focal length of the lens
  A/f = f-number used by photographers to indicate brightness
        of the image at the focal plane.

Thus, animals with sensitive eyes have relatively larger pupil

Table 8.1:   Pupil aperture and f-number of various vertebrates (After Lythgoe, 1979)

Animal	Pupil Aperture (nm)	f-number
Cat (n)	14	0.89[1]
Tawny owl (Strix aluco) (n)	13,3	1,3[2]
Man (d/a)	8	2,1[2]
	7	3,3[3]
Pigeon (Columba livia) (d)	2	4,0[4]

a - arhythmic; d - diurnal; n - nocturnal
1. Vakkur & Bishop, 1963; 2. Martin, 1977;
3. Marshall et al., 1973; 4. Kirschfeld, 1974.

apertures and smaller f-numbers than those of diurnal animals with less sensitive eyes (Table 8.1).

The other method of increasing sensitivity is by the presence of light-reflecting material (tapetum) near the photoreceptor cells in such a way that light which is not absorbed by its initial passage over the photoreceptor cells is reflected back again over them, thus increasing the chance of absorption. Well developed tapeta are usually present in nocturnal animals or those living in very deep, dark or turbid waters (see Chapter 7).

The number of photons absorbed by the visual cells may not always be sufficient for the nervous system to make reliable judgements concerning the nature of the retinal image. Enlargement of the area sampled increases the number of photons absorbed, however, temporal detail suffers. As a consequence fast moving retinal images may not be seen and this is true whether the observer or the display or both are moving (Fig. 8.4). Sampling time (also known as memory time, integration time, or summation time) is estimated by taking advantage of the fact that for periods less than the sampling time an increase in the photon flux can be compensated for by a decrease in the exposure time. Thus up to a certain exposure time sensitivity increases as the flash duration increases but beyond that an increase in flash duration

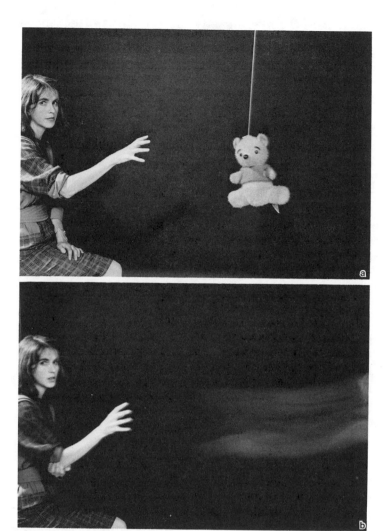

Fig. 8.4: Effect of light intensity on sampling time. The lengthening of sampling time to compensate for lower light intensities results in greater sensitivity and poorer movement perception.

(a)   Photograph taken at 250 lux, 1/60th sec exposure, F-8: the bear, swinging from the string from which it is suspended, is clearly visible.

(b)   Photograph taken at 2,5 lux, 4 sec exposure, F-8:   the bear swinging from the string now appears as a blur. The person swinging it still shows up clearly.

results in no increase in sensitivity. Flicker fusion frequency (FFF)
determinations (see Chapter 2) form a convenient means of
estimating retinal sampling time. Fast-moving, diurnal animals
have fast FFF while slow moving, chiefly nocturnal animals have
low FFF. For human scotopic vision the sampling time is 0,1 sec
while the FFF at near threshold intensities is less than 10 Hz. On
the other hand the retinal sampling time for photopic vision is
0,035 - 0,06 sec and the FFF in bright lights is 50 - 60 Hz (see
Lythgoe, 1979).

Summary

This chapter dealt specifically with visual adaptations for
acuity and sensitivity, however, modifications of any kind is usually
reflected in other aspects. This is well illustrated in Table 8.2
which also serves as a summary of this chapter.

Table 8.2: Rewards and penalties of various visual adaptations
(Lythgoe, 1979)

Feature	Rewards	Penalties
Increase pupil area	Brighter image, better definition	Larger eye or reduced field of view
Increase depth of visual pigment	Better photon capture	Reduced colour discrimination
Yellow filters	Reduce scatter	Reduced sensitivity and spectral range
Summation: Little	Better acuity	Reduced sensitivity
Much	Better sensitivity	Reduced acuity
Memory time: Long	Greater sensitivity	Reduced movement perception
Short	Improved motion perception	Reduced sensitivity
Different receptor types	Colour vision	Reduced sensitivity
Tapetum	Greater sensitivity	Reduced acuity
Screening pigments	Greater acuity	? Reduced sensitivity

9

COLOUR VISION

Light is an electro-magnetic wave characterised by two qualitative factors:brightness and colour. Although both are functions of energy and wavelength, brightness is a function of total energy, while colour is primarily dependent on wavelength discrimination. Traditionally two qualitative aspects of colour have been recognised: hue - the predominant wavelength of a spectral colour; and saturation - the amount of the predominant wavelength in the spectral distribution.

The stimulus to the eye is light and it should be borne in mind that mixtures of coloured lights and coloured pigments (as used in painting) differ. Colour vision is the faculty of the organism to distinguish lights of different spectral qualities. Thus, lights with wavelengths of, for example, 450 nm and 550 nm will appear different to the eye and this difference cannot be eliminated by changes of intensity. In the absence of colour vision, however, these two lights of different wavelengths may be adjusted to produce the same kind of visual stimulus (a certain shade of grey), i.e. lights, regardless of their physical composition, produce the same effect in organisms lacking colour vision. By international convention the three primary coloured lights are: red (700 nm), green (546 nm) and blue (435 nm). These lights when mixed in appropriate quantities can produce white light (Fig. 9.1) or any colour of the visual spectrum. The secondary colours yellow, magenta (violet) and cyan (blue-green) are formed by the pairs of primary colours (red and green; red and blue; blue and green; respectively). Complementary coloured lights are those which when mixed form white light (Fig. 9.1). Thus, for example, yellow (mixture of red and green) and blue are complementary; so are magenta (mixture of red and blue) and green; and cyan (mixture of blue and green) and red.

161

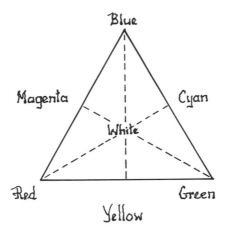

Fig. 9.1: The vertices of the triangle indicate the primary colours, and the sides of the triangle the secondary colours. The combination of a secondary colour and the primary colour opposite it in the triangle (complementary colours) results in white light.

Vision of Monochromats

Receptors having the same spectral sensitivity cannot show qualitatively different responses to lights of different wavelengths. Animals with monochromatic vision may be either rod monochromats or cone monochromats.   These monochromats contain photoreceptors which have a single spectral sensitivity curve (Fig. 9.2).

In the case of the rod monochromats whose retina contains rods only, or at least a retina where the cones do not respond to light (e.g. a normal individual at light intensities below the threshold levels of cones) the spectral sensitivity curve is that of rods (Fig. 9.2). This is explained very simply by the theory that all wavelengths act on rhodopsin, the photosensitive pigment of rods, in the same manner. From this it follows that rods are unable to send coded information about the wavelength of the light acting on them.

The explanation for cone monochromats, however, is not as

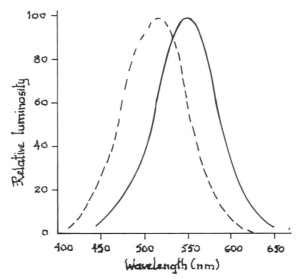

Fig. 9.2: Spectral sensitivity curves of a cone monochromat
(━━) and of a rod monochromat (▪▪▪▪). Maxima of the curves
set arbitrarily at the same level.
(After Pitt, 1944)

simple.   If it is assumed that the cone pigments of the cone
monochromat have all the same spectral sensitivity then the vision
of this monochromat may be explained on similar grounds as the all
rod monochromat.   Thus, three types of cone monochromats might
be expected due to a loss of any two of the three cones.   Cases
which have been studied seem to possess either green or blue cones
only.   Cases of cone monochromatism are extremely rare and it is
unclear if the defect is due to a receptor or a more central
malfunction.   At the very most cone monochromats possess very
rudimentary colour vision, even in regions of the retina which
contain both rods and cones.   The spectral sensitivity curve of the
cones of a cone monochromat is different from that of rods (Fig.
9.2) and is a prima facie case showing that the co-existence of two
types of photoreceptors with different spectral sensitivities is not a
sufficient condition for well-developed colour vision.   In this
instance it is postulated that the nerve fibres from the cone and
rod converge to a single fibre at some level in the transmission
process.   As it is this fibre which is more immediately connected
with the motor centre it follows that the organism cannot respond
in a qualitatively different manner to the stimulation of rods and
cones in various ratios.   Even in the extreme cases in which rods

alone or cones alone are stimulated there will be no difference in the kind of stimulation produced in the common path leading to the motor centre.   Thus it follows that it is possible for cone monochromats to exhibit colour vision if the nervous connexions were arranged differently. Although this is a reasonable suggestion it is unlikely as the high acuity of cone monochromats supports the view that there is a one-to-one connexion of cones to nerve fibres.

Retinal photoreceptors do not send coded nerve messages to the brain about the wavelength of the incident light. Accordingly, when all the receptors have the same spectral sensitivity there can be no colour vision.   The presence of receptors with different spectral sensitivities, although necessary for colour vision, is not by itself a sufficient condition (see: Determination of Colour Vision).

Vision of Dichromats

As may be expected dichromats possess two types of cones with different spectral sensitivity curves (Fig. 9.3). The third cone channel may be defective or altogether absent (Fig. 9.3) thus resulting in only two spectral sensitivity curves (Fig. 9.3). Dichromats may be protanopes (lacking the first, red-sensitive pigment); deuteranopes (lacking the second, green-sensitive pigment); or tritanopes (lacking the third, blue-sensitive pigment) (Fig. 9.4). In these dichromats light of a certain wavelength will stimulate one type of cone to a greater degree than the other, i.e. the ratio of stimulation will differ.   This ratio of stimulation is independent of light intensity.   It is also possible that dichromatic vision may be the result of the fusion of two cone channels.   For example, it is possible for the red and green cone responses to fuse to form a yellow channel but for no output to arise from the red-green colour difference channel.   This may result if the red and green pigments are present within the same cone or, more likely, due to a subsequent central fusion of the two colour channels (Fig. 9.3).   In these dichromats light of two different wavelengths will stimulate these cones in a different ratio but these lights will be mixed such that the cones will respond as if they were stimulated by light of an intermediate wavelength.   Thus dichromats can: 1) respond differently to different lights; and 2) give an identical response to certain lights notwithstanding the fact that they are physically different.

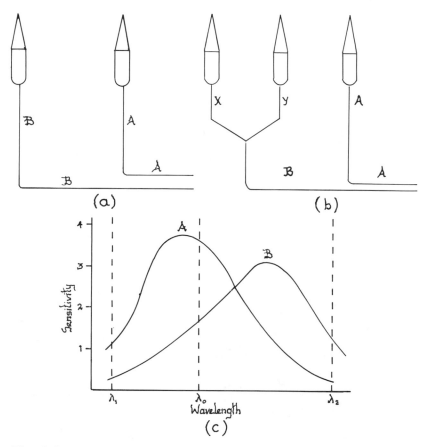

Fig. 9.3: Dichromats may contain only two types of cones (A, B; 9.3a), each with different spectral sensitivity curves (9.3c). Light of different wavelengths will stimulate cone A and cone B in different degrees. Wavelength λ_1 will stimulate A to a greater degree than B, while wavelength λ_2 will do the reverse.
OR
Dichromats may contain three types of cones (X, Y, A) but two of the cone channels (X, Y) may be fused (9.3b) or one may be defective or absent. Thus this individual will respond to colour in the same way as another who possesses only two cone types (9.3c).
(After Pirenne, 1967)

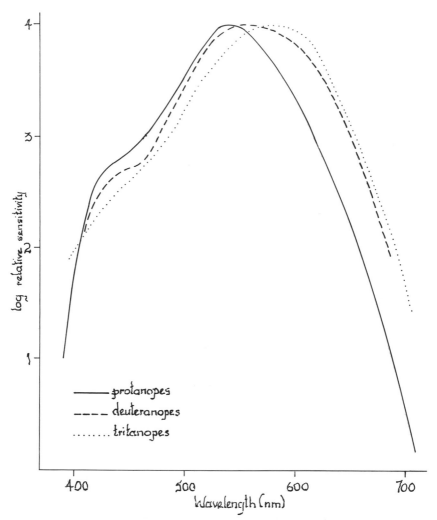

Fig. 9.4: The photopic luminosity function of protanopes (red-blind), deuteranopes (green-blind) and tritanopes (blue-blind). (After Wald, 1964).

Vision of Trichromats

The vision of a trichromat is more complicated. The theory, put forward by Thomas Young in 1802 and later extended by Helmholtz suggested that the retina contains three different kinds of cones, each containing a different kind of light sensitive pigment maximally sensitive in a different region of the spectrum, but nonetheless also sensitive to other parts of the spectrum (Fig. 9.5). The stimulation of each different coloured cone is separately transmitted to the brain where it is then combined to reproduce the outside colours of the world. Microspectrophotometric studies on the retinas of the goldfish, monkey and man showed that there are indeed three types of cones: green (formerly yellow) absorbing (chlorolabe), red absorbing (erythrolabe) and blue absorbing (cynaolabe) (see MacNichol et al., 1973).

The Young-Helmholtz theory, however, has not gone un-challenged. Hering proposed that there are six basic sensations arranged in opponent pairs: black/white, blue/yellow and red/green. One of each pair is thought to drive a catabolic process and the other an anabolic process. Other theories assume that only a single receptor type is needed which would signal colour as well as brightness by an appropriate neural code.

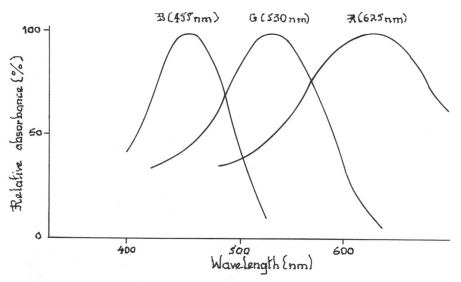

Fig. 9.5: Comparison of goldfish cone absorption spectra based on porphyropsin absorption of Bridges (1967) according to the Dartnall principle. Apsorption spectra of blue sensitive cones (B - peak at 455 nm); green-sensitive cones (G - peak at 530 nm); and red-sensitive cones (R - peak at 625 nm). (After MacNichol et al., 1973)

Recent studies (see Padgham & Saunders, 1975) showed that light appears to be received by three different types of cones, as postulated by the Young-Helmholtz theory, and these are sensitive to the red, green and blue regions of the spectrum. However, the outputs from them appear to be changed into spike discharges and coded before they are transmitted to the brain. This coded information is sent as a luminosity signal receiving inputs from all the types of cones, and as two-colour difference signals (Fig. 9.6). The first colour difference signal is the red versus the green signal which receives inputs from both the red and green cones and then weighs them up before sending the signal which depends upon their selective strengths. The second is the yellow versus the blue signal which acts in a similar way, except that the yellow information is derived by compounding inputs from both the red and the green cones. From this it appears that both the Young-Helmholtz and Hering theories are valid, the first at the receptor level and the second at a later stage in the retina after the signals from the receptors have been coded.

Defects in Colour Vision

Defects in colour vision as apparent in the monochromats and dichromats have been dealt with under their appropriate headings. Trichromats may also exhibit defective colour vision - anomalous trichromats. In this case, although still requiring the three primaries to complete the colour match, anomalous trichromats use quantities of the primaries sufficiently different from the normal trichromat. Consequently the names protanomalous, deuter-anomalous and tritanomalous are used to indicate a reduced sensitivity principally in the red, green and blue regions of the visible spectrum, respectively. Strongly anomalous subjects tend to have colour characteristics similar to the corresponding dichromats and the terms protan, deutan and tritan are often used to include both the corresponding dichromat and anomalous subjects.

Congenital colour defects are more apparent in males than in females as colour vision appears to be associated with the sex (X) chromosome. A female with XX chromosomes will not show colour defects even if one of the X chromosome is defective for colour vision, she will nevertheless be a carrier. A male, on the other hand, with XY chromosomes will be colour defective if his X chromosome is defective (Fig. 9.7).

Besides the inherited defects in colour vision, defects may also be acquired. The excessive consumption of tobacco, alcohol

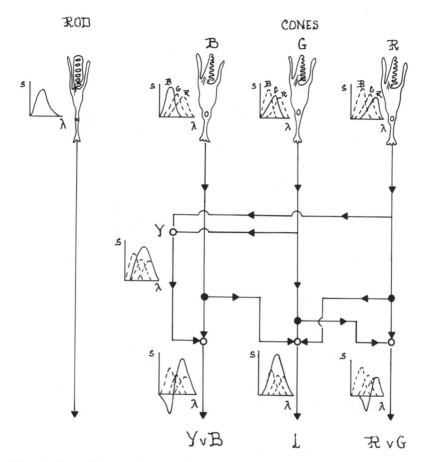

Fig. 9.6: The coding of information in the retina into luminance and colour difference signals. The relative sensitivities of each mechanism (rod, cone) are shown at each stage.

B   -blue cone
G   -green cone
R   -red cone
L   -luminosity
YvB, RvG   -colour difference.
(After Padgham & Saunders, 1975)

and stimulants have also been known to induce the deterioration of colour vision. Ocular diseases such as glaucoma, ocular hypertension and in particular those diseases which affect macular or

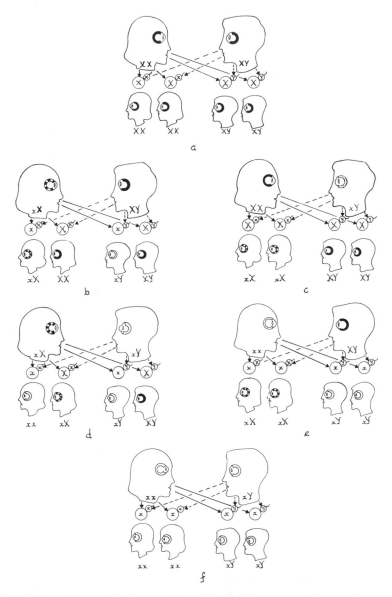

Fig. 9.7: Colour-blindness is sex-linked in man. These figures show how this trait may be transmitted. The solid black retina (XX, XY) indicates normal colour vision; the white retina (xx, xY) indicates red-green colour blindness; while the broken retina (xX) represents the heterozygous condition in the female; these females although exhibiting normal colour vision

central vision have associated colour defects involving normally a deterioration of red-green or blue-yellow discrimination. In addition, aging of the lens may also lead to deterioration of colour vision.

Colour Vision in Animals

Fishes

As far as fishes are concerned no species properly investigated has been shown to be colour blind and the evidence of colour vision in some is very good.

Species which are active near the water surface, where light is bright and spectrally broad, contain the broadest range of visual pigments. This is true for both marine and freshwater species. The carp and the goldfish have been shown to possess trichromatic colour vision. It is interesting to note that the retinal sensitivity of the guppy (Poecilia reticulata), which possesses trichromatic vision, is related to its behaviour (Levine & MacNichol, 1982). The dorsal retina of this fish, onto which is focussed light from below and in front of its visual field, contains the three types of spectral sensitive cones; while the ventral retina, which receives light from the above visual field, contains only green sensitive cones (Fig. 9.8). The male guppy, in order to attract the female, positions itself slightly ahead and below the female so that its image falls on the most colour-sensitive region of the female's retina. The green-sensitive lower retina, on the other hand, is better situated to finding pieces of food silhouetted against the green space light above (Fig. 9.8).

In marine waters, at intermediate depths, the red (long wavelength) light is almost entirely absorbed and species at such depths lack the pigments which absorb red light - their cones being maximally sensitive to blue and green lights. An exception to this is the sea raven (Hemitripterus americanus) which contains cones sensitive to blue, green and yellow-green lights. This is thought to be related to their breeding behaviour. Although spending most of its life at depths of more than 100 metres, during the breeding season (late autumn) this fish moves to shallow waters, here the

---

are nonetheless carriers and can pass the colour-blind trait on to the next generation (b, d).

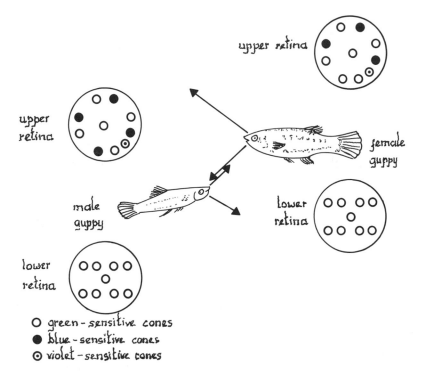

Fig. 9.8: Colour sensitivity of the guppy (Poecilia reticulata).
Cone distribution in upper and lower retinas of the male and
female guppy. See text for further explanations.
(From Levine & MacNichol, 1982)

sexually mature individuals turn yellow, orange and scarlet.   In
addition, after fertilisation, the eggs are deposited on a species of
sponge that is bright orange or yellow (see Levine & MacNichol,
1982).

     Freshwater fishes, other than those inhabiting surface waters,
differ   somewhat   from   their   marine   counterparts.   Thus,   the
freshwater species inhabiting heavily stained waters (e.g. the tiger
barb, Barbus tetrazona; the cichlid fish, Cichlasoma longimanus)
while still possessing three kinds of visual pigments have their
maximum sensitivities in the longer wavelengths of the spectrum.
The bluegill (Lepomis macrochirus), walleye (Stizostedion vitreum)
and piranha (Serrasalmus sp.) inhabit the so called "black waters".
These fishes are active primarily at dawn or dusk near the surface
while   preferring   greater   depths   during   the   day.   Hence   their

spectral environment remains relatively similar throughout the day. These fishes contain few, if any, blue-sensitive cones although they do have green- and red-sensitive cones. The final group of these fishes contains retinas consisting only of rods and green- and red-sensitive cones. They do not have blue-sensitive pigments, and in some species the green-sensitive pigments are also missing; these fishes contain red-sensitive cones only because the dim background space-light is highly red-shifted. Species in this group include numerous catfishes (e.g. Corydoras meyers) and the ecologically similar red-tailed black shark (Labeo bicolor).

Amphibians

Apparently, the tadpoles of the frog (Rana temporaria) are colour blind, while the adults are able to distinguish between red and blue (Birukow & Knoll, 1952). Good colour vision is also claimed for six species of Urodela, while colour blindness was found in three species of toad (Birukow, 1952).

Reptiles

Among the reptiles, lizards have pure-cone retinas and appear to have colour vision. Lacerta agilis and Anolis carolinensis are able to discriminate hues. On the other hand, two species of nocturnal gecko, Hemidactylus turcicus and Tarentola mauritanica, which have pure-rod retinas are colour blind.

Tortoises and turtles probably all have colour vision. Training experiments with three tortoise and one turtle species have shown that they are able to distinguish different hues one from another and from a series of greys (Kries, 1896; Quaranta, 1949, 1952). In addition, as in birds, coloured oil droplets are also present in the sclerad region of certain cone ellipsoids. These oil droplets are considered to act as filters, thereby permitting colour discrimination.

Birds

No one seriously questions that diurnal birds have colour vision. Herring-gull chicks react specifically to the red spot on their parents' bills, while budgerigars recognise the sex of their companions by the colour of the ceres - the male has a blue cere, the female a brown one. It has been shown that males will attack a female whose cere is painted blue and court a male whose cere is painted brown. Similarly, a sexually mature male robin (red breast) will only attack another robin with a red breast, while ignoring the immature male (lacking the red breast). In addition, the domestic fowl appears to enjoy trichromatic vision resembling closely that of man. Trichromatic vision has also been shown for pigeons.

All birds have both rods and cones in their retinas, but the proportions are very different between diurnal and nocturnal species. In addition, oil droplets (red, orange, yellow, yellow-green, colourless) are present in the cones of birds (Fig. 2.4). Nocturnal birds such as owls and nightjars have very few coloured oil droplets and indeed very few cones, however the possibility of trichromatic vision has been demonstrated in the tawny owl (Strix aluco) (Bowmaker & Martin, 1978). Birds which catch insects on the wing also have very few coloured oil droplets as their prime visual task, when feeding, is to detect silhouettes against the background blue light of the sky; coloured oil droplets which reduce sensitivity to blue would make this task more difficult. The diurnal passerine birds, on the other hand, have a high percentage (50% - 80%) of red and orange droplets. This is thought to be related to the vegetarian diet of these species (Bowmaker, 1980); they need the ability to distinguish between different types of foliage and berries.

Coastal birds which feed under water (e.g. shags) and from the surface of the water (e.g. gulls) show variation in the coloured droplets. Gulls have 50% - 80% red and orange droplets. Muntz (1972) suggested that this enhances the bird's ability to see through the water's surface, while Lythgoe (1979) suggested that they have the opposite effect and instead are an adaptation to detect other birds through atmospheric haze. In shags the presence of, only about, 20% red and orange droplets is thought to be an adaptation enabling these birds to detect fish through water where shorter wavelength sensitivity would be advantageous.

Mammals

Mammals with colour vision are rare, only tree-dwelling and fruit-eating species (squirrels and primates) seem equipped for colour discrimination. This is thought to aid them in the acquisation of food; colour vision is not as important to herbivores and carnivores.

The tree shrew which has a pure-cone retina and which is strictly diurnal is able to distinguish red, yellow, green and blue papers from 62 shades of grey between black and white (Tigges, 1963). Investigation on various squirrels (the red squirrel, the American red squirrel, the sousliki or European ground squirrel) with pure-cone retinas showed that they do not have well-developed colour sense, although all indicate some hue discrimination. It is possible that squirrels have only two retinal mechanisms for hue discrimination. Their spectral sensitivity curves show insensitivity to red and two maxima in the green and blue.

Most mammals have rod dominated retinas and some have pure-rod ones. The house mouse, the long-tailed field mouse, the rat, the guinea-pig, the rabbit, the racoon, the polecat, and the cat have all been shown to be colour blind, although some have claimed a poor colour sense for the cat. The ability of a bull to see red is a fable - it will just as well charge at a differently coloured muleta. The horse may have rudiments of colour vision, and although some (Colvin & Burford, 1909; Samoiloff & Pheophilaktova, 1907) claim that dogs do possess very weak colour vision the dog is generally thought to be colour blind. A dog trained to "fetch" a coloured ball (e.g. red) will fetch a ball of similar brightness (i.e. same shade of grey).

Determination of Colour Vision

The possession of a retinal mechanism for analysing wavelength differences apparently does not necessarily mean that the owner of the retina has colour vision. Thus some differential wavelength sensitivity has been demonstrated in the cat, the rat and the guinea-pig but behaviour experiments indicate that neither of these animals has colour vision (see Tansley, 1965).

The most satisfactory method of discovering whether or not an animal has true colour vision is by training experiments. These are tedious and time-consuming and it is very important that they be properly controlled. It must be established beyond all doubt that the animal under training is making its discrimination on the basis of hue alone and not by other cues such as smell, hearing, touch or position. It is also vital to know that the animal's choice is not really on the basis of brightness instead of colour. If an animal is trained to go to a green target and to avoid a red one it is necessary to adjust the intensities of the two stimuli so that they appear equally bright to the animal. In order to do this a knowledge of its spectral sensitivity curve is necessary. If the green and red stimuli are of equal physical intensity the red one will usually appear darker to an animal because its retina is less sensitive to the long wavelengths. It is not even enough to equate the intensities so that they look equally bright to the human eye, for the animal's spectral sensitivity curve is not necessarily the same as the human one. It is desirable to establish the spectral sensitivity curve before proceeding to test hue discrimination. This can be done by training positive to the brighter of two targets after which it is relatively easy to establish which parts of the spectrum look brighter and which darker by exposing different coloured stimuli in pairs. It is then possible to train to a target of a given colour and to match this with various others so that they will appear equally bright to the animal in question. By this means it will be possible to determine whether there is discrimination on the basis of hue alone and, depending on how many colours are tested, get some idea of the efficiency of hue discrimination throughout the spectrum. Such elaborate experiments are rarely done. It is more usual to train the experimental animal to a given colour and then to present this colour paired with a series of greys ranging from black to white. If enough greys are used in the range and the animal always makes the correct choice it is certain that this choice is made on the basis of hue and not on the basis of brightness. Then the animal has colour vision.

Training experiments are usually only possible in animals of relatively high intelligence and which will become sufficiently tame to be trained. In cases where this is not easy or even possible, use has been made of the optomotor reaction. For such experiments a hollow rotating cylinder is painted inside with vertical stripes of two alternate colours or of one colour and a grey. If two colours are used, it is necessary once again to know the spectral sensitivity curve so that the colours may be equated in brightness for the animal. This method has been severely criticised on the grounds that it will be so difficult as to be virtually impossible to get an absolute equation between brightness of the stripes and that this will suggest colour vision where there is actually none. If there is no optomotor reaction the inference is that the alternating stripes look identical to the animal. When the optomotor reaction is used negative results may be more reliable than positive ones.

Another method which has been used is to colour the animal's food, either by dyeing or by illumination with coloured lights, and to see which colour it seems to prefer. There are several objections to this procedure. There is absolutely no way of knowing whether the choice is made on the basis of brightness or of hue. Besides, the animal may ignore food of one colour not because it cannot see it but because food is never that colour in nature! Erroneous conclusions were reached about the hen's sensitivity to blue light as a result of using this method. Grain were illuminated with spectral lights and it was found that the seeds lying under the blue end of the spectrum were not taken. It was concluded that the hen's eye is not sensitive to blue because they apparently could not see the blue seed (Hess, 1912). Later work in which hens were trained to differently coloured grains showed that they are sensitive to blue after all (Walls, 1942).

Some workers believe that if an animal shows a Purkinje shift it must have colour vision. Their argument assumes that cone vision is always coloured vision. Although it is true that colour vision appears to be associated with cones and light adaptation we do not know that all predominantly cone eyes possess colour vision (e.g. various squirrels). A Purkinje shift only demonstrates that the retina in question possess two types of visual cell with different spectral sensitivity curves, one used predominantly in the light-adapted state, the other in the dark-adapted state. It proves nothing either way about whether colour vision is present or not. Some pure-cone eyes, which show no Purkinje shift, may well have colour vision.

Besides training experiments colour vision tests may be carried out by retinal densitometry (see Chapter 3). Here, a beam of light is projected into the fovea and the amount reflected measured by a sensitive photo-electric cell. The amount of light absorbed by the visual pigment can be measured by comparing the amount of monochromatic light reflected by the unbleached or dark-adapted eye with that reflected by the bleached or light-adapted eye. If this is carried out at selected wavelengths absorption curves can be obtained. If two pigments are present a complex function is obtained but if one is present the function is relatively simple and its form will be independent of the wave-length of the bleaching light. Microspectrophotometry (MSP) may also be used to determine the presence of colour vision based on the spectral properties of visual pigments located on photoreceptor outer segment membranes. This method, which combines micro-scopy (to identify the cell type under examination) and spectro-photometry (to determine the presence and concentration of the visual pigment), is discussed in Chapter 3. Other techniques for detecting colour vision are based on electrophysiological measure-ments using electrodes placed externally to the eye and brain. The electroretinogram (ERG) monitors retinal functions while the electronencephalogram (EEG) monitors more central visual processes. At present, however, ERG and EEG are mainly restricted to research applications.

10

VISUAL TRANSDUCTION

Recent advances in biochemical and physiological techniques have introduced fresh insights into the mechanisms that regulate the transduction of light energy into electrical impulses in vertebrate photoreceptors. Most of these studies were carried out with rods, however cones are also thought to operate along similar lines.

The vertebrate rod photoreceptor is a classic example of a cell which is functionally dependent on an internal transmitter. The site of phototransduction is the outer segment. In the rod, the outer segment consists of membranous discs which, except for a few basal discs, are structurally, osmotically and electrically isolated from the plasma membrane. Visual pigment molecules which are located primarily on these discs absorb the photons, yet it is the plasma membrane which exhibits a transient suppression of ionic permeability. This in turn leads to graded hyperpolarisation of the cell, which eventually reaches the synaptic terminal whence it is then transmitted to second order neurones for further processing. In this chapter the proposed mechanisms which bridge the gap between photon absorption and permeability of the cell are considered.

The exact nature of the light-sensitive current in vertebrate photoreceptors has yet to be fully understood. The selectivity of the channel, which may be a pore or a carrier, is still controversial. Studies have not unequivocally established that sodium is the only ion whose permeability through the plasma membrane is modulated by light. However, under natural circumstances, it is the primary event responsible for the hyperpolarisation of the visual cell. Contrary to the above, events which occur from the time of photon

179

absorption to changes in ionic permeability of the plasma membrane are still not explicit.

There is general agreement that the light-sensitive permeability of the rod outer segment (ROS) plasma membrane is regulated by transmitter(s) which relate(s) changes occurring at the site of photon absorption on disc membranes to the sites governing membrane conductance on the plasma membrane. Furthermore, as several channels are closed following the absorption of a single photon, there must be an intervening amplification step.

Any model for excitation must generate the relationship between light intensity and receptor response. This entails that the transduction process must be initially linear with light intensity and subsequently saturated (Fig. 10.1), i.e. it should satisfy the following equation:-

$$a = a_{max} \; I/(I+\sigma)$$

where:
a   - light response amplitude
a_{max} - maximal response amplitude
I   - light intensity
σ - light intensity that results in a half maximal light response.

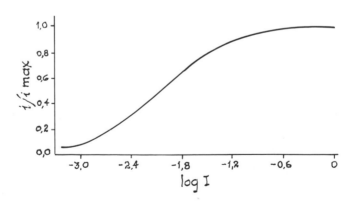

Fig. 10.1: Voltage-clamp intensity-response relationship for a vertebrate rod.   Normalised amplitudes of light-suppressed currents as function of log flash intensity.
(After Bader et al., 1979)

For both vertebrate and invertebrate photoreceptors there is a latent period of about 100 msec between the time a dark-adapted photoreceptor is exposed to a brief dim flash of light and the occurrence of the photoresponse. Under these conditions the duration of the light response is approximately 1 sec. Both latency and duration of response vary with intensity and duration of the light stimulus. Two mechanisms are currently favoured. The first suggests that calcium ions are involved; while the second suggests that the reactions may be enzymatically regulated (Fig. 10.2). The presence of calcium and the enzymes regulating cyclic nucleotide levels (cyclase, phosphodiesterase) in photoreceptor outer segments have been demonstrated ultracytochemically (see Athanassious, 1983).

A key feature of the internal transmitter hypothesis is that it provides high gain to account for the high sensitivity of the rod photoreceptor. In order to meet the requirements of a transmitter the substance proposed must undergo a significant concentration change when the photoreceptor is exposed to light, and that photoreceptor excitation is dependent on its change in concentration - it is this change which elicits photoreceptor excitation.

Calcium Hypothesis

The actual role of calcium in phototransduction is as elusive today as it was when initially proposed as the intracellular messenger mediating excitation (Yoshikami & Hagins, 1971). According to this hypothesis, in darkness ROS contain much higher intradiscal calcium (2 - 9 mM) than the cytosol (10^{-8} - 10^{-16} M). In light, calcium released from discs increases the cytosolic free calcium which in turn closes the sodium channels (Fig. 10.2). Illumination releases intradiscal calcium into the cytosol in rods; whereas in cones, calcium from the extracellular space provides a nearly inexhaustible source of calcium (1 mM) for release into the intracellular compartments (lamellae of cone outer segments).

Rise in cytoplasmic calcium in ROS is illustrated by the increase in calcium concentration in the interstitial space surrounding these photoreceptors when excised living retinas are exposed to light. The intracellular change of calcium concentration was estimated to be of the order of $2,1\pm0,8\times10^4$ $Ca^{2+}.R*^{-1}.Rod^{-1}$. Although this figure may appear high, it underestimates the changes in calcium concentration occurring within the cell. Nevertheless, the amplitude and kinetics of extracellular calcium changes, as well as their dependence on the receptor

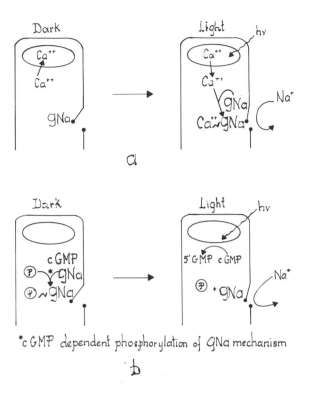

Fig. 10.2:   Two models linking photon absorption to sodium permeability of the plasma membrane based on :-
(a)   calcium hypothesis - light-induced calcium released from discs combines with the sodium gates of the plasma membrane thus inhibiting sodium conductance.
(b)   cyclic nucleotide hypothesis - light activates a phospho-diesterase enzyme which lowers the cyclic nucleotide level, this in turn causes dephosphorylation of the sodium gate which leads to closure of the sodium channel and hence decrease of sodium conductance.
g Na -sodium gate.
(After Hubbell & Bownds, 1979)

potential, suggest that these changes are intimately involved in transduction.

Bound calcium of the ROS discs forms more than 99% of stored calcium but the binding site is unknown. Phosphatidylserine, a major component of ROS membranes, is a prime candidate for the binding site. This implies that phosphatidylserine is located primarily on the inner surface of the disc membrane. However, this is not supported by the transbilayer distribution of phospholipids in disc membranes and the low charge at the inner surface of the disc membrane (see Kaupp & Schnetkamp, 1982). In addition, the mechanism of transdiscal calcium transport (intradiscal $\rightleftharpoons$ cytoplasm) is unknown. Finally, the most important question remains unresolved:- Is the store of intradiscal calcium involved in the regulation of cytosolic calcium? Not all investigators (Liebman, 1978; Szuts, 1981; Szuts & Cone, 1977) were able to detect calcium release from discs. Thus, for calcium to remain the internal transmitter of phototransduction, it was proposed that the light-sensitive calcium pool resides within the cytosol in a bound form (Szuts, 1981; see also Athanassious et al., 1984). Cytoplasm is known to contain substances which bind calcium (e.g. nucleotides and protein-bound phosphates), but the actual magnitude of this bound cytosolic calcium is unknown. This modified calcium hypothesis suggests that the light-sensitive cytoplasmic pool is only slightly larger than the free pool which, in the frog, is of the order of 10^{-6} M or $0,001\ Ca^{2+}.R^{-1}$ (Hagins & Yoshikami, 1974).

The strongest evidence in favour of the calcium hypothesis is the large efflux of this ion when ROS are illuminated. However, conclusions about the role of this calcium efflux must await the location of the source of this calcium within the ROS.

Negative Transmitter Hypothesis

The second theory advanced to explain the process of visual transduction is based on the enzymatic control of the proposed transmitter - cyclic guanosine 3',5'-monophosphate (cGMP). This theory is also known as the "Negative Transmitter Hypothesis" because it is the reduction of cGMP in rods following illumination which initiates the closure of the sodium channels of the plasma membrane and thus its hyperpolarisation (Fig. 10.2).

Enzymes immediately involved in the control of cyclic nucleotide (cNMP) levels are the synthesising (cyclase) and hydrolysing (phosphodiesterase, PDE) enzymes.

$$NTP \xrightarrow{\text{cyclase}} cNMP \xrightarrow{\text{PDE}} 5'\text{-NMP}$$

(3',5'-NMP)

+

pyrophosphate

Thus, regulation of either cyclase (inhibition) or PDE (activation), or both of these enzymes can bring about a decrease in cNMP levels. When this theory was first advanced by Bitensky and Miller in 1970 (see Bitensky et al., 1981) it was suggested that adenosine 3',5'-monophosphate (cAMP) was the cyclic nucleotide involved, and that it was the inhibition of adenylate cyclase, by light, which regulated the cAMP levels. Subsequent investigations revealed that although the cNMP level in ROS is photo-regulated, it is the cGMP which is involved, and rather than cyclase it is the cGMP-PDE which is activated by light (see Miller, 1981).

Most of these studies were carried out with rods. In cones cAMP levels are not only higher than cGMP levels, but it also appears to be modulated by light. This led to the suggestion that cAMP may function in the same way in cones as cGMP does in the physiological events which occur in rods following photon absorption (see Farber, 1981).

The fundamental aspects of the cNMP hypothesis are illustrated in Fig. 10.3. Light activates rhodopsin (**R***) which then complexes with a protein (**E.GDP**) called transducin (Stryer et al., 1981) or G-unit (Bitensky et al., 1981) to form a transient complex (**R*.E.GDP**) which proceeds to exchange its nucleotide for GTP. As **R*** has a higher affinity for **E.GTP**, in the presence of **E.GDP**, **R*** dissociates from **E.GTP** to bind preferentially to the former. The activated protein (**E*.GTP**) removes the inhibition on PDE thus forming the active form of phosphodiesterase (**PDE.E*.GTP**) which hydrolyses cGMP at the rate of 10^5 cGMP molecules $sec^{-1}.R*^{-1}$ (Stryer et al., 1981). Restoration of the dark state occurs via hydrolysis of the GTP bound to PDE and phosphorylation of **R*** by rhodopsin kinase.

One of the major criticisms against the role of cGMP in visual transduction is the relative inefficiency of a negative transmitter. It is argued that the plasma membrane is less likely to detect a decrease in cGMP concentration, which in the dark is about 40 - 90 μM in ROS, than to detect the presence of a few hundred calcium ions above the background (cytoplasm) which is

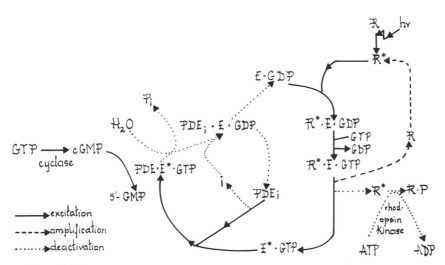

Fig. 10.3: Diagrammatic representation of the negative transmitter hypothesis. (See text for details)

postulated to be zero (see Sorbi, 1981). However, the plasma membrane should be able to detect fast and pronounced decrease in cGMP concentrations in the microdomain of excitation if the transmitter synthesis in the surrounding space is slow compared to PDE activity (i.e. hydrolysis faster than synthesis). Another point advanced against the cGMP theory is that its reduction is not rapid enough, significant decrease being noted only after 3 - 5 sec of the light stimulus (Gordis et al., 1977; Govardovskii & Berman, 1981; Kilbride & Ebrey, 1979). In order to be effective in the closure of sodium channels cGMP should decrease within the latency of the photoresponse i.e. within 100 msec of the stimulus. However, it is argued that the function of cGMP in excitation is highly compartmentalised and that small changes in this cGMP pool is below the level of detection of current techniques.

Thus, the cGMP hypothesis, as with the calcium hypothesis, still needs to be clarified. Data currently available indicate that cGMP metabolism is intricately involved with photoreceptor function, however, the precise role played by it in phototransduction must await verification.

M. A. ALI AND M. A. KLYNE

Calcium and cGMP

It is highly unlikely that the complex processes of visual transduction are mediated by any single reaction. Thus the question now arises:- How is it possible to unite the data which favour calcium as the internal transmitter to those which favour cGMP? The calcium and cyclic nucleotide systems may both be intricately involved; e.g. the diffusion coefficient for the ROS longitudinal spread of both excitation and adaptation is within a factor of two of that for both calcium and cGMP (Yau et al., 1981).

Three basic schemes are immediately suggested (see Lipton & Dowling, 1981).

Scheme I: Calcium and cGMP both serve as intracellular mess-engers which function independently of each other in the regulation of membrane potential.

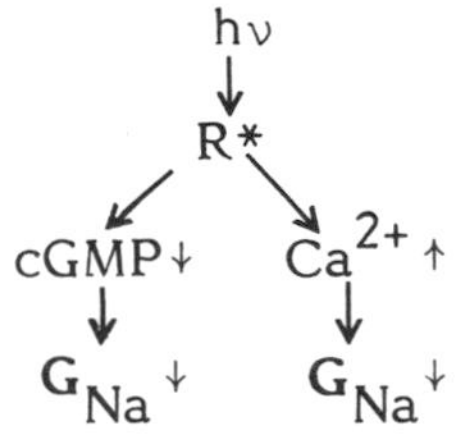

$$h\nu$$
$$\downarrow$$
$$R*$$
$$\swarrow \qquad \searrow$$
$$cGMP\downarrow \qquad Ca^{2+}\uparrow$$
$$\downarrow \qquad \qquad \downarrow$$
$$G_{Na}\downarrow \qquad G_{Na}\downarrow$$

where G_{Na} is the sodium current

Scheme II: Calcium and cGMP serve as dual, sequential mess-engers, i.e. alteration in the level of one influences the other's level which in turn regulates the sodium current.

$$h\nu \rightarrow R* \rightarrow Ca^{2+}_{cyto}\uparrow \rightarrow cGMP\downarrow \rightarrow G_{Na}\downarrow \qquad (a)$$

$$h\nu \rightarrow R* \rightarrow cGMP\downarrow \rightarrow Ca^{2+}_{cyto}\uparrow \rightarrow G_{Na}\downarrow \qquad (b)$$

Scheme III: Only one of these substances (calcium or cGMP) serves as the intracellular messenger, while the other modulates the concentration of the messenger.

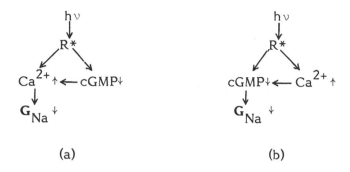

(a)   (b)

Of the three schemes, Scheme I seems unlikely. Cohen et al. (1978) showed that the decrease in cytosolic calcium causes a dramatic increase in levels of cytosolic cGMP, thus indicating that these substances are inter-related. It is therefore apparent that both calcium and cGMP are coprimary and complementary factors in the process of visual transduction. In invertebrate photoreceptors sodium channels are transmembrane proteins containing binding sites for which calcium and sodium may compete antagonistically. When sodium is bound to the site the channel is open for sodium conductance, however, when calcium is bound to the site the channel is closed for sodium conductance. A similar arrangement has been proposed for vertebrate photoreceptors (Schnetkamp, 1980). This hypothesis may be considered in conjunction with cGMP effects on calcium binding sites; cGMP is thought to decrease the binding site affinity for calcium and increase its affinity for sodium. Thus, in the dark when cGMP concentrations are elevated sodium binds to and opens the channels (Fig. 10.4). In

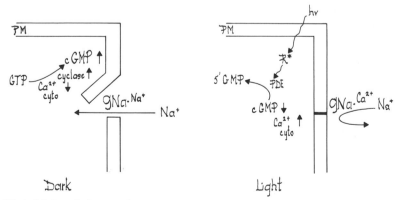

Fig. 10.4: Schematic representation of the calcium and cGMP hypotheses of visual transduction. (See text for details)

light, cGMP concentrations in the microdomain fall because of light activated cGMP-PDE, and calcium binding to the channel is favoured, thereby switching the channel to the closed conformation (Fig. 10.4). Moreover, guanylate cyclase appears to be modulated by calcium - when calcium activity is diminished this enzyme is stimulated and serves to restore the normal cGMP concentration in ROS.

The above would tend to favour Schemes IIb and IIIa. Quick-freezing of retinas by Kilbride and Ebrey (1979) indicate no significant change in cGMP concentration, in ROS, after 1 sec of bright illumination. This result tends to favour Scheme IIIa. More recently Kilbride (1980) found that cGMP levels fall much faster (15 X) in retinas incubated in low calcium Ringer's solution than in normal Ringer. A similar observation was made earlier by Woodruff and Bownds (1979).

In summary, current data indicate that both calcium and the cyclic nucleotide cascade along with rhodopsin are involved in the

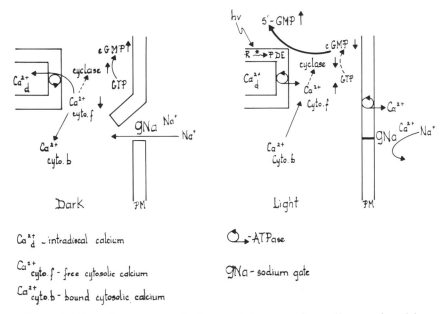

Fig. 10.5: Summary of the calcium and cyclic nucleotide hypotheses of visual transduction. (See text for details)

process of phototransduction whereby light absorption leads to decreased sodium permeability of ROS membranes (Figs. 10.5, 10.6). Photo-activated rhodopsin communicates with cGMP-PDE

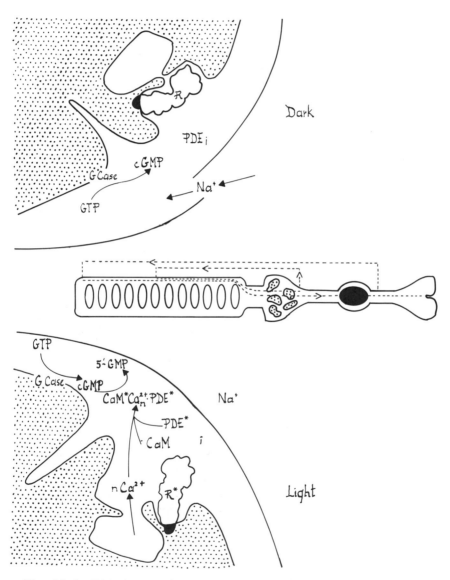

Fig. 10.6: Diagrammatic representation of rod disc and plasma membrane and the events of phototransduction.

then hydrolyses cGMP thus leading to its decline. On the other hand, photo-activated rhodopsin induces an increase in free cytosolic calcium ($Ca^{2+}_{cyto.f}$). Both the decrease in cGMP and the increase in free cytosolic calcium lead to the decrease of the sodium dark current of the ROS plasma membrane. Light is known to cause a release of calcium from ROS of the intact retina into the intracellular space while cGMP decreases calcium binding to discs by 25% (see Miller, 1981). With time/darkness cGMP recovers through the inhibition of cGMP-PDE (caused by the degradation of photolysed rhodopsin, and/or activation of guanylate cyclase (GCase) brought about by the lower calcium levels). The lower free cytosolic calcium results from the conversion of free to bound cytosolic calcium ($Ca^{2+}_{cyto.b}$) or transport of cytosolic calcium into the intradiscal space via a calcium-ATPase pump. Lower free cytosolic calcium weakens its competition for the sodium gates (g_{Na}) on the plasma membrane; sodium then binds to these sites and opens the channels. The plasma membrane potential is thus returned to its dark level.

At a recent Dahlem conference on "The molecular mechanisms of photoreception" (25-30 November 1984, West Berlin) cGMP emerged as the most favoured messenger of phototransduction; while calcium is thought to function in the adaptation process (see Lewin, 1985). It was also postulated that cGMP exerts its effect by direct interaction.   In the dark, the sodium channels on the plasma membrane are thought to be maintained in an open position by the high levels of cGMP in rods and that exposure to light initiates rapid hydrolysis of this cyclic nucleotide thus resulting in closure of these channels. The inability to detect changes in cGMP levels is attributed to:-   i) limitations of current methods to detect the changes; ii) presence of two pools of cGMP – bound and free, the latter being the "active" form but present at very low levels; iii) photostimulation of guanylate cyclase activity leading to synthesis of cGMP, thus hydrolysis of this substance by cGMP-PDE results in an apparent stable level of cGMP while a photo-initiated increase in turnover is maintained. Therefore, although the present trend is towards cGMP as being **the** messenger of visual transduction this subject is far from resolved. There were some participants at the conference who believe that cGMP does not provide answers to the whole story and that other components and parallel pathways may yet be uncovered; e.g. inositol triphosphate has been proposed as a potential messenger in photoreceptors.

11

PROCESSING BY THE CENTRAL NERVOUS SYSTEM

Light absorption by photopigment in a retinal photoreceptor (rod or cone) causes the cell membrane to hyperpolarise. This potential change is then transmitted electronically to synapses on both bipolar and horizontal cells. In turn, the bipolar cells transmit a graded electrical signal to the ganglion and amacrine cells with which they are in contact. In the ganglion cells action potentials are generated and these pass along the optic nerve and tract to the lateral geniculate nucleus and the visual cortex (Fig. 11.1). In the retina lateral interactions are provided by the horizontal and amacrine cells. Generally, the number of fibres in the optic nerve approximate the number of retinal ganglion cells. In primates and birds this number is high while in various amphibians and fishes it is relatively small. The visual pathway from retina to cortex consists essentially of six types of neurones or nerve cells; of which three are in the retina (photoreceptors, bipolar cells, ganglion cells), one in the lateral geniculate nucleus, and two in the cortex (complex and simple cortical cells) (Fig. 11.1). Nothing very mysterious is occurring, but it is nevertheless difficult to fully comprehend the parts and how they are integrated into a whole.

Optic Nerve, Chiasma and Tract

Axons of retinal ganglion cells form the optic nerve which is part of the central nervous system. In lower vertebrates most of these fibres are thin and sparsely myelinated; while in the advanced teleosts and terresterial vertebrates the fibres are heavily myelinated. The convergence of nerve fibres, before emerging behind the eye, forms the optic disc or papilla which is the blind spot in the visual field (Fig. 1.1).

191

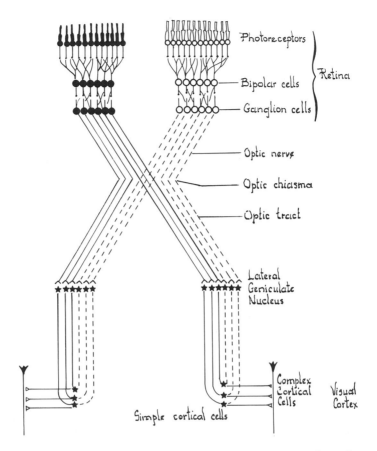

Fig. 11.1:   Schematic representation of the visual pathway, from retina to visual cortex, illustrating the basis of binocular vision.   In man roughly half of the fibres of the optic nerve remain uncrossed at the optic chiasma.   These ipsilateral (uncrossed) fibres from the outer part of the retina of one eye join with the contralateral (crossed) fibres from the inner part of the retina of the other eye and they travel together to the lateral geniculate nucleus where they are segregated into layers.   The fibres that emerge from this body carry an input from both eyes, they then converge on single neurones in the cortex.
(From Pettigrew, 1972)

        The optic nerve fibres form the chiasma by decussating below the floor of the diencephalon.   This decussation is complete or almost complete in all submammalian vertebrates and in some lower mammals. In the frog, lizard, snake and duck a small number of fibres remain ipsilateral (uncrossed) in the optic chiasma. In advanced mammals, particularly primates, the decussation is partial (in man 50 per cent of the fibres of the optic nerve are uncrossed). Only fibres from the nasal side of the retina cross; those from the temporal side remain ipsilateral. The optic chiasma does not contain neurones or synapses. The part played by decussation in image reversal is illustrated in Fig. 11.2.

The optic tract is the continuation of the optic nerves posterior to the chiasma (Fig. 11.1). As the result of partial decussation, in advanced mammals, the optic tract contains fibres from both optic nerves in these species. In man, as in other primates, the optic tract contains an almost equal number of fibres from each eye (Fig. 11.2). An intermediate condition occurs in other mammals; fibres from the contralateral eye still predominate in each optic tract. In the rat, 90 per cent of the optic nerve fibres decussate in the chiasma (Fig. 11.2). In submammalian vertebrates, most optic tract fibres terminate, without decussation, in the optic tectum (Fig. 11.2); a few fibres or collaterals pass to the thalamus. In mammals almost all fibres end in the thalamus, although, even in man, some fibres terminate in the superior colliculus.

The basal optic root is a small bundle of thin fibres that separates from the optic tract in terresterial vertebrates, passes around the cerebral peduncle in mammals, and terminates in the basal optic nucleus (ectomammillary body), associated with the medial part of the substantia nigra. A few fibres of the basal optic root end in the lateral reticular formation of the tegmentum of the midbrain and in the oculomotor nucleus. The basal optic root arises in the contralateral eye. A few optic nerve fibres also project to the hypothalamus in some submammalian species.

Optic Tectum

The optic tectum (superior colliculus in mammals) is a laminated structure which forms the roof of the midbrain in all vertebrates. It is absent in amphioxus and is poorly differentiated in myxinoids, while having, relatively, the largest size in teleostean fishes.

Besides being the primary visual centre in all vertebrates, except mammals, the optic tectum also functions as the major correlative centre of non-optic exteroceptive impulses in lower

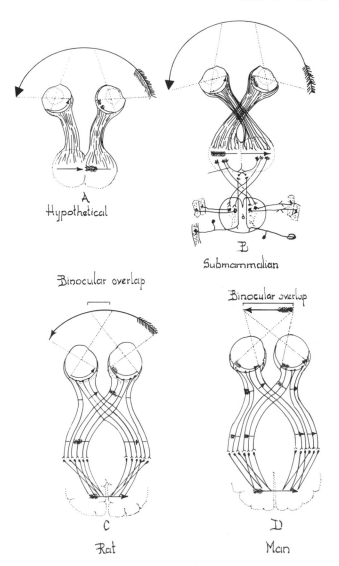

A
Hypothetical

Binocular overlap

B
Submammalian

Binocular overlap

C
Rat

D
Man

Fig. 11.2: Schematic representation for the decussation of the optic nerve fibres in providing image reversal and binocular vision. Failure of optic nerve fibres to decussate results in an illogical projection in the optic tectum. The hypothetical condition (A) of complete lack of decussation is not found in any vertebrate. Total decussation of optic nerve fibres (B) allows full panoramic vision, a condition found in sub-mammalian vertebrates. Partial decussation of the optic

vertebrates.   It is partly because of the latter function that the tectum remains well developed in species with small eyes and poor vision.

The early embryologic condition of the optic tectum of higher vertebrates is similar to that of urodelan amphibians. It consists of a central layer of neurones and a superficial layer of fibres, the latter being stratified with afferent fibres peripheral to the efferent paths. The optic tectum of the lamprey differs from that of other vertebrates in possessing a superficial layer of ependyma, but the lamination of the optic tectum is particularly well organised relative to the other parts of the brain.

A pattern common to most vertebrates is:-

1.   An external white layer (stratum opticum) composed of afferent fibres of the optic tract and brachium tecti (geniculotectal tract).

2.   The main receptive layer for terminal fibres of the optic nerve and the spinotectal and bulbotectal pathways is the intermediate gray and white layer (stratum fibrosum et griseum superficiale; stratum lemnisci). It is involved in relaying somatic sensory information for correlation with visual impulses. Reciprocal connexions with pars lateralis of the substantia nigra also occur.   This layer is better differentiated in teleosts and reptiles than in elasmobranchs and anuran amphibians due to complete migration of neurones during development.   Non-optic afferent projections are important in lower vertebrates while in mammals they are insignificant.

3.   The deep gray layer (stratum griseum centrale or profundum) is a cellular lamina with dendrites extending superficially into

---

nerve fibres (the mammalian condition) requires overlap of terminating fibres in the secondary ascending visual pathway to reconstruct images in a logical retinotopic pattern and superimpose corresponding images from the two eyes on the visual neocortex. An animal's overlap of the two visual fields is proportional to the percentage of uncrossed fibres in the optic chiasma. As animals evolved with eyes occupying a more frontal position this percentage tends to increase. In lower mammals (e.g. rat, C) most optic nerve fibres will decussate but in higher species (including man, D) nearly half project ipsilaterally.
(From Sarnat & Netsky, 1974)

the external white layer and intermediate gray and white layers. These cells are the final efferent neurones of the optic tectum, and the axons form the underlying fourth layer.

4.   The deep white layer has many commissural fibres connecting the optic tecti of the two sides, as well as other decussating tectal fibres.

5.   The superficial neurones of the periaqueductal gray matter have dendrites extending into the optic tectum as far as the external white layer.

Mammals have similar tectal lamination as lower vertebrates. In addition, they have, superficial to the external white layer, one more layer of neurones covered by a zonal layer of slightly myelinated fibres. These superficial white and gray layers in mammals are associated with the development of the visual neocortex. The zonal layer is composed of fibres from the cortical region corresponding to the frontal eye field, and from the auditory and visual associative neocortex of the temporo-parieto-occipital region. The pathway is called the external corticotectal tract. An internal corticotectal tract from the lateral surface of the occipital lobe (areas 18 and 19 of Brodmann) terminates somato-topically in the intermediate gray and white layer of the tectum in mammals. In man, these heavily myelinated fibres are the largest afferent projection to the optic tectum. In reptiles, only a few of such fibres occur. The corticotectal fibres may be related to movements of eyes in visual tracking.

The medial bulbotectal and spinotectal tracts emerge from the deep white layer of the optic tectum, curve ventrally around the periaqueductal gray matter, and decussate ventral to the oculomotor nuclei in the dorsal tegmental decussation (dorsal fountain decussation of Meynert), before proceeding caudally, ventral to the medial longitudinal fasciculus. Fibres have a direct tectocerebellar part but mammals have tectopontine fibres for the relay of visual impulses to the cerebellum via the pontine nuclei. Corticopontine fibres also arise in the primary and associative visual areas of the cerebral cortex in mammals.

Pretectal Area

Homology of the pretectal area in different vertebrates is difficult to determine. The group of neurones usually designated as the pretectal area is anterior to and continuous with the middle gray layer of the optic tectum. Afferent fibres of the pretectal area are from the optic tract and the lateral geniculate body. The retinopretectal fibres in the mouse, rat, rabbit and tree shrew are predominantly crossed although a few fibres also terminate in the pretectal nuclei on the same side as the eye of origin.   The pretectal area has efferent connexions with the optic tectum, lateral geniculate body, nucleus rotundus (pulvinar) of the thalamus, the Edinger-Westphal nucleus and tegmental reticular formation of the midbrain.

Dorsal Thalamus

The dorsal thalamus (or simply thalamus) is a large diencephalic structure receiving ascending fibre projections from many systems including the visual system of lower vertebrates and mammals.   This led to the recognition of homology of many thalamic nuclei in different vertebrates and a uniform nomenclature was proposed by Ebbesson (1972) (Fig. 11.3; Table 11.1).

The lateral geniculate body is important in relaying optic impulses to the visual cortex in man and other mammals, however, it is also well developed in many lower vertebrates lacking a neocortex typical of mammals. Although small, it persists in the blind species of fishes, while a thalamic structure similar to the lateral geniculate body is well developed and even laminated in many teleosts. In most vertebrates, the lateral geniculate body consists of ventral and dorsal nuclei.   The ventral nucleus (well developed in teleosts) is not only a synaptic centre between the optic tectum and the tegmentum of the midbrain, but also receives fibres from the optic tract. In mammals, the ventral nucleus is large in rodents but decreases in size as one ascends in phylogeny, such that in man only a few neurones remain as the pregeniculate nucleus. The tectogeniculate pathway is called the brachiumtecti and is prominent in teleosts.   The brachium of the superior colliculus persists in man but is mainly an afferent pathway to the optic tectum, rather than efferent.

The dorsal nucleus of the lateral geniculate body is largest in mammals, while in reptiles it is less well developed, though distinct.   The efferent fibres of the dorsal nucleus of the lateral geniculate body form the optic radiation or geniculocalcarine tract to the neocortex in mammals.   Geniculate connexions with the forebrain are lacking in teleosts, but anuran amphibians have a few fibres from the posterior part of the lateral geniculate body to the lateral wall of the cerebral hemisphere. In reptiles and lower mammals, the lateral geniculate body is large. In reptiles, the ventral nucleus extends the length of the diencephalon. In the

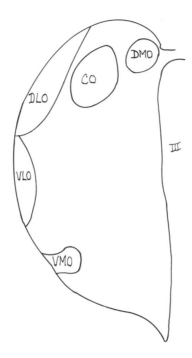

Fig. 11.3:   Highly schematic representation of topologic
positions of some optic nuclei found in all vertebrates.
DMO - dorsomedial optic nucleus; DLO - dorsolateral optic
nucleus; CO - central optic nucleus; III - third ventricle; VLO -
ventrolateral optic nucleus; VMO - ventromedial optic nucleus.
(From Ebbesson, 1972)

opossum, the dorsal nucleus predominates and forms the entire
lateral wall of the thalamus.   The lateral geniculate body has
reciprocal connexions with the thalamic nuclei, particularly with
the overlying pulvinar, in all mammals.   This nucleus of the
posterior part of the thalamus is present in carnivores and
ungulates, however it is well developed only in primates.   The
nucleus rotundus of submammalian vertebrates is the homologous
counterpart of at least the mammalian pulvinar.

In addition to descending projections from the tectum,
ascending fibres occur in all vertebrates, being prominent in
reptiles, birds and mammals. Tectogeniculate fibres terminate in
both ventral and dorsal nuclei of the lateral geniculate body. The
dorsal nucleus projects to the general cortex or primordial

Table 11.1: Proposal for new nomenclature of thalamic nuclei of the visual system. Such a classification enables the identification of homologous nuclei by common names in all classes of vertebrates (After Ebbesson, 1972)

	Dorso-medial optic nucleus (DMO)	Dorso-lateral optic nucleus (DLO)	Ventro-lateral optic nucleus (VLO)	Ventro-medial optic nucleus (VMO)	Central optic nucleus (CO)
Elasmobranchs	Pretectal area	Lateral geniculate nucleus	Ventro-lateral optic nucleus	Unknown	Lateral geniculate nucleus
Teleosts	Dorso-medial pretectal nucleus; dorsolateral thalamic nucleus	Uncertain	Uncertain	Ecto-mammillary nucleus; nucleus of the posterior accessory optic root	Nucleus rotundus; prethalamic nucleus
Amphibians	Pretectal area	Dorsal thalamus	Visual part of ventral thalamus	Ecto-mammillary nucleus	Visual part of dorsal thalamus
Reptiles	Postero-dorsal nucleus	Dorso-lateral geniculate nucleus	Ventral geniculate nucleus	Ecto-mammillary nucleus	Nucleus rotundus
Birds	Uncertain	Dorso-lateral anterior complex	Ventral geniculate nucleus	Ecto-mammillary nucleus	Nucleus rotundus
Mammals	Pretectal area; pretectal nucleus; olivary pretectal nucleus	Dorsal nucleus of lateral geniculate body	Ventral nucleus of the lateral geniculate body; pregeniculate nucleus	Medial terminal nucleus of basal optic root	Pulvinar; posterior lateral thalamic nucleus

neocortex of amphibians and reptiles, and to the calcarine or primary cortex of mammals. These ascending geniculotelencephalic projections have been found also in elasmobranchs.

A second ascending pathway from the optic tectum also occurs in reptiles, birds and mammals (Fig. 11.4). The diencephalic centre of this pathway is the nucleus rotundus. Unlike the lateral geniculate body, the nucleus rotundus (pulvinar) does not receive direct retinal fibres of the optic tract. In contrast to the tecto-geniculo-cortical pathway that terminates in the primary visual

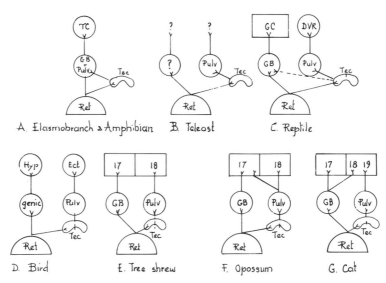

Fig. 11.4: Schematic representation of variations in visual pathways among vertebrates, based on studies using Nauta's technique. (A) The shark has a single thalamic centre of the visual system (GB and Pulv) to which both retinal (Ret) and tectal (Tec) fibres project. This thalamic nucleus discharges to one nonlaminated telencephalic centre (TC). The arrangement in amphibians is similar, although the thalamotelencephalic projection is not well understood. (B) Teleosts have direct retinal connexions to a thalamic centre different from the centre in which tectal fibres terminate (Pulv). Further ascending pathways to the telencephalon are unknown. (C) Reptiles have a well-developed geniculate body (GB) of the thalamus that receives retinal and sparse tectal fibres and projects to the laminated general cortex (GC) of the telencephalon. A second visual pathway ascends from tectum to

cortex, the tecto-pulvino-cortical pathway in lower mammals projects to the nonstriate secondary visual neocortex. The two ascending systems partly overlap in some mammals but are separate in the tree shrew. In advanced mammals, the pulvinar receives some tectal fibres as well as short connexions from the lateral geniculate body. The ascending visual pathways in vertebrates are schematically represented in Fig. 11.4.

Visual Centres in the Telencephalon

The traditional concept is that the optic tectum is the principal visual centre in submammalian vertebrates and that its function shifts to the telencephalon (cerebral cortex) in mammals. Recent studies (Graeber et al., 1973; Graeber & Ebbesson, 1972) suggest that vision is a telencephalic function that evolved early in at least some vertebrates, including mammals, and that if cephalisation of vision occurred as an evolutionary change, it did so long before the first primitive mammal appeared. A telencephalic centre is found in the shark, whereas, in teleosts the optic tectum is the principal visual centre. An explanation of this is that elasmobranchs are not ancestral to teleosts and that the primitive visual system included a telencephalic region as its highest centre. Teleosts departed from this arrangement by developing the tectum as a highly specialised visual structure that incorporated the telencephalic visual function of the vertebrates. The optic tectum is relatively larger in teleosts than in other vertebrates.

---

nucleus rotundus or pulvinar (Pulv), then to a nonlaminated telencephalic structure of the dorsalventricular ridge (DVR). (D) Birds have the greatest separation of two ascending visual systems, terminating in hyperstriatum (Hyp) and ectostriatum (Ect). Both of the latter structures are of telencephalic origin and are probably homologous with mammalian neocortex. (E) The tree shrew has the greatest separation of visual systems among mammals, with no overlap in neocortex. (F) The opossum has two ascending visual systems with overlap in area 17. (G) The cat has an arrangement similar to the opossum but with overlap in areas 18 and 19. Area 17 is the primary visual, or calcarine, cortex; and areas 18 and 19 are associative visual cortex. The extent of the ascending visual system in man is unknown.
(Modified from Ebbesson, 1972)

Visual function in the telencephalon of amphibians and reptiles is still lacking, as is the importance of secondary visual pathways through the pulvinar to the neocortex of mammals. The optic tectum did not atrophy or disappear with the evolution of higher visual centres in the telencephalon of advanced vertebrates. This suggests that the ascending pathways have a specific, and probably unique, function in the visual system of mammals. In the tree shrew, tectal lesions result in inattention to visual stimuli and impairment of visual identification of objects. In contrast, the cerebral cortex was thought to inhibit incorrect responses to the total visual information received (Jane et al., 1972). In man, inattention or neglect and visual agnosia are associated with lesions of the neocortical parietal lobe. In reptiles and, especially, in birds direct retinal projections to the dorsal nucleus of the lateral geniculate body (dorsal anterior nucleus) occur in addition to the tectothalamic pathways. Birds lack the neocortex, but the highly differentiated, unique structures of the corpus striatum probably incorporate the reptilian primordium of the neocortex and function similarly. Thus the highest visual centres in birds are in the telencephalon, a condition similar to that found in mammals. Elasmobranchs and some other lower vertebrates also may have a telencephalic visual system more similar to that of man than was previously recognised.

Evolution of the Mechanisms of Vision

The visual system of lower vertebrates (e.g. frogs) is organised for the recognition of a few stereotyped patterns. In the frog, discrimination of food is determined by size and movement. This may be related in part to the lack of a macula or fovea in the retina of the frog. The brain of the frog is activated by four patterns of visual images (sharp edges with contrast; curved edge of a dark object; movement of edges; focal or general dimmings produced by movement or rapid darkening within the total visual field). A separate group of fibres in the optic nerve deals with each detectable pattern. These fibres are mixed within the optic nerve. The retinal field is projected as four separate layers of nerve endings in the optic tectum, and each layer corresponds to one of the four basic functions.

The arrangement of the neocortex serving vision in mammals differs somewhat from that of the optic tectum (superior colliculus) of either mammals or lower vertebrates. Mechanisms of visual perception in the dorsal nucleus of the lateral geniculate body and calcarine cortex, however, are reminescent of the less complex condition in the optic tectum of the frog. The visual mechanism in the cat and the monkey are similar although greater precision is found in the latter. The mechanism of vision in man is probably similar.

Individual neurones of the calcarine cortex specifically respond to stimulation by white light in restricted areas of the retina. In mammals, the calcarine cortex is subdivided into discrete regions or columns. Neurones within each column respond to stimuli in the same axis within the retinal receptive field. Cortical columns may be round or oval in cross-section with the majority being elongated and narrow. The diameter is about 0,5 mm in the cat and is smaller in the monkey. In some parts of the calcarine cortex the columns are arranged in a regular manner with a progressive gradual shift in the orientation of the columns. In other regions of the cortex the adjacent columns are randomly oriented with respect to one another. The smallest receptive fields are near the fovea centralis, the fields tend to be larger in the periphery of the retina. Each cortical column receives projections from several simple receptive fields as well as from more complex fields in which the response to a stimulus cannot be predicted from the arrangement of excitatory and inhibitory regions. Neurones of the more complex fields tend to be in laminae II, III, V, VI and are binocularly activated in the monkey. Cells of the simple receptive fields are generally deep in layers III, IV-A and IV-B. About 80 per cent of all neurones of the calcarine cortex of the cat are influenced independently by the two eyes. In binocularly influenced neurones, the two receptive fields which have the same orientation of axis and are situated in corresponding parts of both retina are stimulated simultaneously.

The superior colliculus of mammals has an organisation similar in some respects to that of the calcarine cortex; vertical columns of neurones have specific axes of orientation. Little is known about mechanism of vision in birds. Many, particularly birds of prey have extremely sharp visual acuity. They probably perceive images as do mammals rather than the limited number of specific patterns to which the frog responds.

Vision is particularly important to maintain proper orientation in flight. In birds, as in man, the visual system predominates over the vestibular as the primary mechanism of spatial orientation, although all animals are capable of adapting to blindness by greater reliance upon vestibular, auditory and proprioceptive cues.

Binocular (Stereoscopic) Vision

Most animals, including mammals, have laterally directed
eyes on the sides of the head. This arrangement allows very little
overlap of the visual field of each eye and this allows for
panoramic rather than binocular vision (Fig. 11.2B). Primates
(from the tarsier and lemur through to man) on the other hand have
eyes directed forward with overlap of all but the most temporal
parts of the visual field. The overlap of the two visual fields is
associated with the degree of decussation of the optic nerve fibres
in the chiasma (the overlap being proportional to the percentage of
ipsilateral fibres). Each side of the brain thus subserving one side
of the composite visual field.

Binocular vision, the fusion of images seen at a slightly
different angle with each eye, provides a means of locating objects
in space - a visual aptitude called stereopsis or solid vision. The
overlap of the visual fields of primates and, to a lesser extent, of
cats and other mammals allows for stereoscopic vision. In man,
depth perception is effective only for objects up to a few feet away
as at greater distances the difference in visual angle between the
two eyes becomes insignificant. Beyond this, depth perception is
based on the relative difference in size of objects and visual
experience.

Partial decussation serves to bring the optic nerve fibres
together in the brain. At the first way station (the lateral
geniculate nucleus) the inputs from the two eyes are carefully
segregated into layers. The more binocular overlap the animal has,
the more obvious is the layering. This segregation has been
confirmed by physiological recordings which showed that a neurone,
or nerve cell, in a given layer of the lateral geniculate nucleus can
be excited by light stimuli following on one eye only (Fig. 11.5).
The segregation is reinforced by inhibitory connexions between
corresponding neurones in adjacent layers. At the level of the
visual cortex of the brain, however, single neurones do receive
excitory inputs from both eyes.

It is uncertain if the second macula of birds, or even if the
single macula of birds such as the owl (with frontal eyes) results in
binocular vision. Overlap of visual fields and fusion certainly
occur, but it is still speculative that the optic tectum or visual
hyperstriatum of birds can fuse the two images stereoscopically as
the neocortex does in mammals. Many lizards move each eye
independently of the other, or converge to focus both eyes
simultaneously on the same object. Different neural pathways are

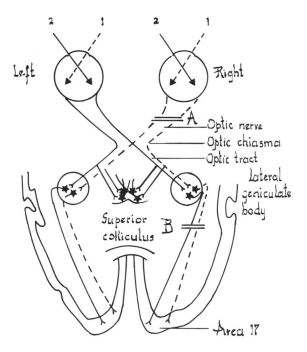

Fig. 11.5: The visual pathways. When looking straight ahead,
light from objects in the right visual field (arrows numbered 1)
reaches the left halves of the retinas. The reverse being true
for the left visual field. The collaterals from the visual path
(to the superior colliculi for reflexes) are really separate
fibres and not branches of true visual fibres. Cutting the optic
nerve at **A** causes complete blindness in the right eye. A
lesion at **B** however causes blindness in the left half of each
field of vision (Arrows numbered 2).
(From Gardner, 1975)

needed, however for panoramic and stereoscopic vision (Fig. 11.2).

Processing of Colour Vision

In order to process colour information, a cell in the central
nervous system must receive inputs from more than one cone type.
However, this is not the sole factor, the unit may well be
extracting movement rather than colour information from the
cones. This confusion arose from the reference to cones as colour
receptors and the use of colour names for the various cone types.

This was further amplified by the discovery of midget bipolar cells (Polyak, 1941) which picked up information from one cone and fed it to one ganglion cell - assuming no lateral interactions among horizontal and amacrine cells.   Cones rather than being 'colour receptors' are 'light receptors', each responding to every wavelength, intensity, shape, whether moving or stationary. Thus, it has been suggested (DeValois, 1973) that they be referred to as:-

L-cone -cones   containing   **long**-wavelength   absorbing   pigment
        λ_{max} - 570 nm (red);
M-cone -cones containing   **medium**- wavelength absorbing pigment
        λ_{max} - 540 nm (green);
S-cone -cones   containing   **short**-wavelength   absorbing   pigment
        λ_{max} - 445 nm (blue).

In higher vertebrates, retinal projections to central structures is up four fairly well-defined paths:- the lateral geniculate nucleus (LGN) and from there to the striate cortex; the superior colliculus; the pretectal area; and the accessory optic nerve. However, most of the information available on the central mechanisms of colour vision comes from studies on the activity of cells at just one non-retinal locus - the LGN.   Thus, very little can be said about the transformation of colour information beyond the LGN, nevertheless, much of the processing of colour information does appear to take place before the cortex. The participation of the geniculo-striate path in colour processing in the primate central nervous system is illustrated by defects in colour discrimination as a result of cortical lesions in monkeys - no similar loss resulted from destruction of the superior colliculus. In the tree shrew (Tupaia glis) the situation is quite different. The animal was still capable of colour discriminations before and after a total striate lesion.

The LGN, of primates, contains cells which respond differently to colour rather than to luminance difference - opponent-cell responses, similar to the opponent S-potentials found by Svaetichin. In the primate, there appears to be two separate colour systems (DeValois et al., 1966). The RG system (+R-G and +G-R cells) contains cells which exhibit peak responses to red and green, and cross from excitation to inhibition above 560 nm. The other is the YB system (+Y-B and +B-Y cells) and it contains cells which cross from excitation to inhibition below 560 nm and which show peak responses to yellow and blue (Fig. 11.6). In addition to the above four varieties of spectrally opponent cells, other cells found in the LGN of the macaque do not give spectrally opponent responses, but rather respond in the same direction (excitation or inhibition) to light of all wavelengths (Fig. 11.6). These cell types correspond very closely to the types of retinal outputs which Hering (1878) postulated to account for colour appearances (Fig. 9.7).

Spectrally opponent cells form a large proportion of the LGN of the macaque monkey (70% - 80%). These cells have also been found in the squirrel monkey (Saimiri sciureus) and spider monkey (Ateles); although their number is smaller especially in the latter. The ground squirrel (Citellus mexicanus), a dichromat, possesses spectrally opponent cells of the YB variety only. The cat, with its limited colour vision, also contains spectrally opponent cells, however, they form only about 3% of the cells of the LGN.

Cone Inputs to LGN Cells

RG cells (+R-G, +G-R) of the LGN of the macaque receive inputs from L- and M-cones. One of the cone types being excitatory and the other inhibitory to these opponent cells. Thus, the firing of these cells does not reflect the degree of excitation/-inhibition produced by the L-/M-cones but rather the difference between the amount of excitation and inhibition produced at each spectral point by the two different cone types. The point at which these cells show maximum excitation is thus not 570 nm (λ_{max} for L-cone) but beyond 640 nm; the wavelength at which the difference between the excitation from the L-cone and the amount of inhibition from the M-cone is maximal (Fig. 11.7). Correspondingly, maximum inhibition is not to light of 540 nm (λ_{max} for M-cone) but to light around 520 nm; the wavelength at which the difference between the amount of inhibition from the M-cone and the amount of excitation from the L-cone is maximal (Fig. 11.7). Thus, although RG cells receive inputs from cones maximally sensitive to 570 nm and 540 nm (greenish yellow), they show maximum responses of opposite types to 640 nm (red) and 520 nm (green).

The cone input into the YB cells (+Y-B, +B-Y) is uncertain. One input is clearly from S-cones, but whether the other is from L-cones or M-cones (or both) is uncertain. Wiesel and Hubel (1966) reported that +Y-B cells receive inputs from S- and M-cones; while DeValois (1965) and Abramov (1968) believed that these inputs come from S- and L-cones (Fig. 11.7). A summary of cone inputs into the LGN of the macaque monkey is given in Fig. 11.8. Anatomical, psychophysical and physiological data indicate that rod inputs are also transmitted to the chromatic system in the primate. However, it is unlikely that rods make much of a contribution under photopic conditions because of interactions in the pathway. Besides, the

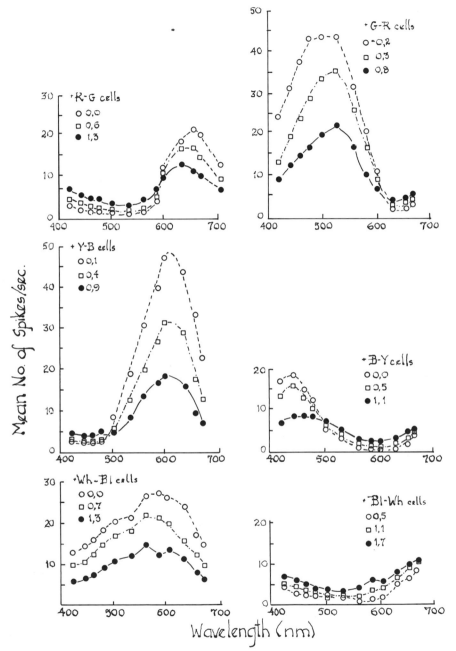

Fig. 11.6:   Average responses of LGN cells.   Plots of the

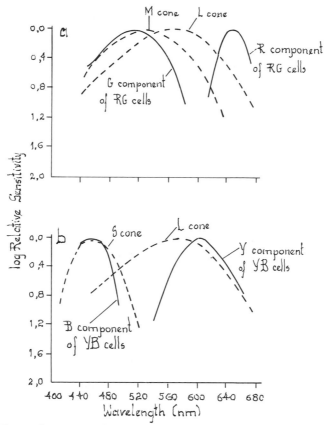

Fig. 11.7: Cones and opponent colour cells. Spectral absorption curves of macaque and human, and the corresponding opponent cells:-

a - L and M cones, and R and G components of the RG opponent cells.

b - S and L cones, and B and Y components of the YB . opponent cells.

solid line - components of opponent cells; dotted line - cones. (After DeValois, 1973)

---

average response rates of macaque LGN cells of four spectrally opponent and two non-opponent cell types. The three curves in each case are the responses to different luminance levels, the neutral densities used being indicated. (From DeValois et al., 1966)

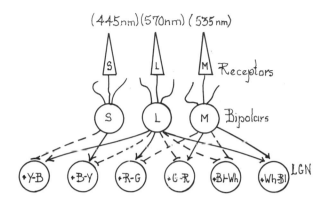

Fig. 11.8: Model of the connexions for colour vision up to the LGN. Inputs of light receptors into four colour and two achromatic channels are shown. Spatial organisation of receptive fields and lateral connexion have been omitted. (After DeValois, 1973)

contribution of rods to colour processing is apparently negative, it tends to desaturate the colours which would otherwise be seen.

Relation to Visual Behaviour

An individual with normal colour vision sees that different parts of the spectrum have different colours under neutral adaptation conditions. Subjects when asked to identify flashes of light by colour names (red, yellow, green or blue; or modified by another colour name from the same four e.g. yellow-red, blue-green, etc.) gave the response shown in Fig. 11.9. This result is comparable to the responses of macaque LGN opponent cells to flashes of light of different wavelengths (Fig. 11.9). Thus, it is apparent that reasonably good agreement exists between psycho-physical and physiological data. Furthermore, the appearance of these close relationships at the LGN suggests that little further processing of colour information per se occurs later in the visual pathway. The data (Fig. 11.9) are, however, incomplete especially at the shorter wavelengths.

Other examples of the relationships between opponent cells in the monkey and colour receptors of man with normal colour vision can be seen in chromatic adaptation studies (Jacobs & Gaylord, 1967) and the Bezold- Brücke phenomenon (Boynton & Gordon, 1965; DeValois et al., 1966).

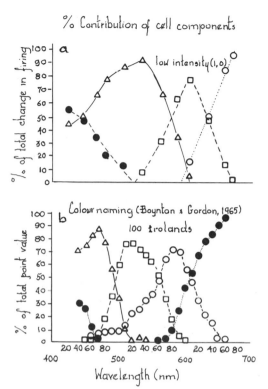

Fig. 11.9: Colour names and opponent cell activity. Comparison of colour names given to different wavelengths (bottom - data from Boynton & Gordon, 1965) with the activity rates of each of the four LGN spectrally opponent cell types (top) Cell types in **a** o: +R-G; □: +Y-B; △: +G-R; ●: +B-Y. Colour names in **b** ● red; o yellow; □ green; △ blue. (From DeValois, 1973)

Behavioural studies indicate that for man and macaques the region around 570 nm is very desaturated relative to the spectral extremes and that the absolute saturation discrimination thresholds are also very similar for these two species. In physiological tests, the spectrally non-opponent cells were found to discriminate among equal luminance lights of varying purity. On the other hand, spectrally opponent cells are very sensitive to purity differences. Responses of +R-G cells to lights of different purities at each of several different wavelengths is illustrated in Fig. 11.10. Similar tests of other cell types indicate that the +B-Y cells can discriminate saturation differences very well in the very short

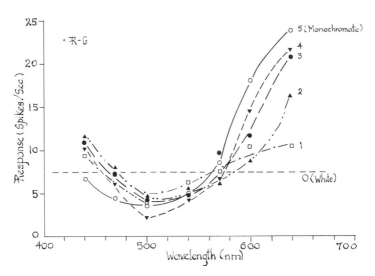

Fig. 11.10:   Responses of +R-G cells to lights of different
purity (saturation).   At each wavelength, a shift was made
from a white light to one of five white-monochromatic
mixtures (of equal luminance). Curve 5 is pure monochromatic
light; curve 4 a slightly desaturated spectrum, etc. It can be
seen that at long wavelengths the +R-G cell's responses were
systematically related to the amount of red in these red-white
mixtures.
(From DeValois & Marrocco, 1971)

wavelengths; and the +G-R cells show relative good saturation
discrimination in the greens.   However, none of the cell types
discriminates saturation differences very well in the yellows.
These data can quantitatively account for the saturation discrimination function seen behaviourally in macaques Fig. 11.11.

Wavelength Discrimination

A person with normal colour vision can readily discriminate
between different wavelengths of light equated for photopic
luminance.   This ability is not uniform across the spectrum.   One
can discriminate small wavelength differences in the yellow-orange
and in the blue-green parts of the spectrum, but only larger
differences in the green and toward either spectral extreme.   The
same holds true for macaque monkeys.

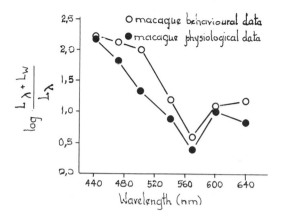

Fig. 11.11: Comparison of saturation discrimination by macaque monkeys and macaque LGN opponent cells. From data compared under three different adaptation conditions (neutral, red and green adapting lights), obtained for each opponent cell type, one can determine the purity level required for a criterion firing level at each wavelength from each cell type. Assuming the animal's behaviour is determined by the cell type which best discriminates at each wavelength, one obtains values plotted in solid dots. The open circles are from psychophysical tests of the ability of monkeys to choose between white and desaturated coloured lights.
(From DeValois & Marrocco, 1971)

Contrast and Similitude

Colour seen at a certain point in space is not only dependent upon the stimulus conditions but also on the stimulus configuration in the surrounding regions and what existed there at a previous time. These interactions are of two different sorts in two different directions and have been termed contrast and similitude. Simultaneous contrast refers to the fact that a surround of one colour or brightness tends to induce into a neighbouring region the opposite colour and brightness (opposite in terms of opponent organisation). Similitude effects are effects in the opposite direction to contrast. Similitude effects refer to the stimulus circumstances under which a surround of a particular colour and brightness induces not the opposite colour and brightness (as in colour effects) but the same colour and brightness into the neighbouring region. The brightness induction effect has also been referred to as assimilation or the Bezold spreading effect.

Summary

In primates, the LGN projects completely to the striate cortex. In the macaque (and most likely in the human visual system) some 70% - 80% of the cells of the LGN transmit colour information. However, what happens to that information once it reaches the cortex is still virtually unknown. Further changes may occur:-
a) -Some unknown interaction must effect the separation of the black-white and colour information being carried by the spectrally opponent cells.
b) -The outputs of the various spectrally opponent cells may be differenciated from each other to produce cells with extremely high spectral selectivity.
c) -Cells of a particular spectrally opponent variety but receiving from different retinal areas may be combined to form coloured-line detectors.
d) -Cells which detect lines of different colours may be combined to form cells which detect lines regardless of colour (although) it is colour information which allows the lines to be detected initially).
e) -Interactions over long distances may occur to provide colour contrast.

12

VISUAL ILLUSIONS

Vision is an active process. The image on the retina is essentially two-dimensional, yet the world is perceived as three-dimensional. Retinal images are but patterns in the eye - patterns of light and dark shapes, with areas of colour - however we do not see patterns, we see objects. Retinal images have no clear boundaries, yet they give the presence of separate, distinct objects; this is brought about by perception. Thus, perception can be thought of as the reading of non-sensed characteristics of objects from available sensory data. It involves a kind of problem solving and is governed by our basic knowledge of objects. We not only believe what we see, to some extent we see what we believe. However, perception can go wrong in many ways, and when this happens visual illusions result. These illusions are of great interest to psychologists.

There is a large number of illusory phenomena, but not all have been regarded with equal interest or subjected to equally intense investigation. In general, they are due to special properties of the figures perceived in conjunction with special characteristics of the visual functions as a whole, including brain processes. Generally the mechanisms underlying them are far from being clearly understood, and may be very complex. Visual illusions may be classified into broad categories; e.g. those that result from size/shape distortion, movement and brightness/colour.

Size/Shape Distortion

Size/shape distortions or illusions are varied, however, they are extraordinarily consistent. They are very much the same every time and are similar for almost all observers. In the more common distortion-illusion figures some lines appear too long or short, others bent, while still others appear to be displaced from their true positions (geometric illusions). Other distortion-illusion figures include ambiguous forms or paradoxes.

Geometric Illusions

These are relatively simple line drawings whose physical dimensions of size, shape or direction are generally misjudged. These errors can be as great as 30 percent or even more - large enough to be a serious problem in practice. They are interesting because, despite their uncomplicated composition, they are difficult to explain. Five of the more common geometric illusions are given in Fig. 12.1. The vertical-horizontal (Fig. 12.1a), Ponzo (Fig. 12.1b) and Müller-Lyer (Fig. 12.1c) illusions are all illusions of size. Here, two drawn features in each of the figures are measurably equal, yet they appear unequal in size.

Arrow 'heads' and 'tails' of the Müller-Lyer illusion are thought to give perspective cues to depth. They have been suggested to represent corners (Gregory, 1970). The flat projection of the Müller-Lyer illusion figure on paper and the image on the eye while looking at an actual corner (arrow tails - inside corner of a room; arrow heads - outside corner of a building) are exactly the same. Thus, the Müller-Lyer illusion figure is thought to trigger the depth scaling system, in this case incorrectly as the figure is two dimensional. Variations of the Müller-Lyer illusion (Fig. 12.2) show that the corner explanation of Gregory (1970) is limited. Rather, it has been suggested (Day, 1972) that the long and short components of the Müller-Lyer illusions are separate illusions. The first is determined by the size of the attachments while the second is determined by the inner space defined by the inner portions of the attachments (Fig. 12.2). The components of the Müller-Lyer illusions are essentially distance stimuli, which under normal visual conditions assist in the preservation of size constancy. Thus, it is essentially similar to other illusions in which the size of the adjacent elements is the principal determinant of the effect. Similarly the Ponzo illusion gives the same projection as parallel lines (e.g. railway). The upper bar appears larger than the lower (Fig. 12.1b), although they are the same length, due to convergence setting 'Constancy Scaling' which is appropriate in the normal three-dimensional world. Here perspective is presented on a flat plane of the picture (Fig. 12.3) and so the compensation, normally giving size constancy is inappropriate. Both these illusions (Müller-Lyer, Ponzo) are illusions of size, and many cues to distance

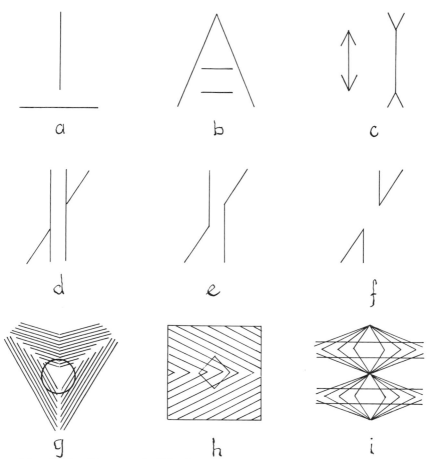

Fig. 12.1: Geometric illusions.

a   -Vertical-horizontal illusions. The two lines are of the
     same length, yet the vertical appears longer.

b   -Ponzo's illusion. The horizontal parallel lines are of
     equal length, yet the top member appear longer.

c   -Müller-Lyer's illusion. Both vertical segments are of
     equal extent yet the one bounded by arrow 'heads'
     appears shorter than the one bounded by arrow 'tails'.

d-f -Poggendorff's illusion. An illusion of misalignment when
     two diagonal lines which lie along the same straight no
     longer appear colinear. Note colinearity decreases with
     angle size - compare e and f.

g-i -Orbison's (g, h) and Hering's (i) illusions. The true shape
     of geometric figures (g - circle, h - square, i - parallel
     lines) appear distorted because of their context.

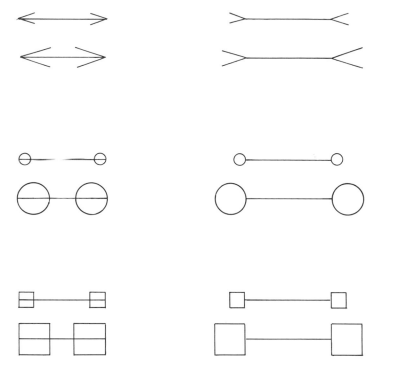

Fig. 12.2: Variations of MÜller-Lyer illusions demonstrating the limitation of the 'corner' theory for the explanation of this phenomenon. The length of the horizontal lines is similar in all instances. On the left, the length of the horizontal line is determined by the inner space defined by the inner attachments - hence the larger the attachments the shorter the apparent length of the horizontal line. On the right, the size of the attachments determines the apparent length of the horizontal line - the larger the attachments the shorter the line appears and vice versa.

including accommodation, convergence, overlay elevation, texture gradient, element size and frequence alone or in combination can contribute to the maintenance of a degree of size constancy (Day, 1972).

The other illusions in Fig. 12.1 are illusions of orientation. In the Poggendorff illusion, two diagonal lines which lie in the same straight line appear to deviate from their path (Fig. 12.1d-f). In these instances it is postulated that acute angles are over

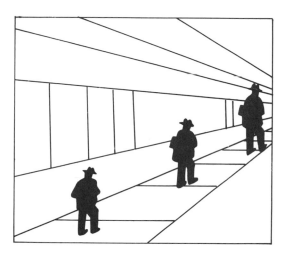

Fig. 12.3: The three silhouettes of the man are identical in size, yet they appear different when seen within their context. (From Bloomer, 1976).

estimated, there being a possible neurological basis for such distortions in the cortex (Burns & Pritchard, 1971; Chiang, 1968). The 'acute angle' hypothesis may be over generalised, but it cannot be dismissed as a possible factor in the genesis of geometrical optical illusions where figures are made to appear distorted because of their context (Fig. 12.1g-i). Ganz (1966) advanced another hypothesis for the explanation of these geometrical illusions. His principle is based on lateral inhibition which he states can account for figural after-effects even though the test and inspection figures are shown at different times. Ganz (1966) then goes on to argue that such phenomena exist even more strongly when contours are presented simultaneously (e.g. in geometrical illusions). Thus progressive displacements of portions of the 'figure' by the 'background' bars due to lateral inhibition could account for these illusory shape distortion of the figures.

There is however, one characteristic which all geometric illusions share i.e. they can be verified by simple measurements (length, angle, radius).

Ambiguous Forms

Generally, the external world has a certain permanence or reliability, however, there may be alternative ways of seeing objects which are genuine and which appear similar to everyone. They may be described as reversible, improbable or multistable. Not all these terms are interchangeable but they all refer to visual displays that elicit from the observer two or more clearly different interpretations. These interpretations may be due to depth and object ambiguity.

There is always an infinite number of possible three-dimensional shapes which will give the same projection on a flat plane. The best known example is the skeleton cube (Necker cube) which is drawn without perspective so that no surface is indicated by a size difference as nearer or further than the other (Necker, 1832). The information conveyed by the figure of the cube (Fig. 12.4) is insufficient for decision making, and the brain never arrives at a definite conclusion. Thus, the skeleton cube is seen in spontaneously reversing depth. The same depth reversibility can also be seen in the solid representations of objects - e.g. cubes, staircase (Fig. 12.5).

Ambiguity in depth is only one form of ambiguity. There is also object ambiguity, here the mind is uncertain as to what is represented by a picture or even if a picture is representing anything at all (e.g. abstract art and the ink blot personality test).

Objects appear as separate entities if they can be distinguished from their surroundings. Contours and differences of texture or colour help, but often boundaries of objects are not

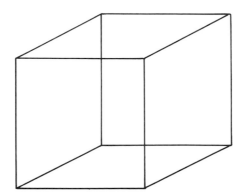

Fig. 12.4: This is a plane projection of a cube as seen from a great distance. There is no perspective size change and the figure is seen in spontaneously reversing depth.
(Necker, 1832)

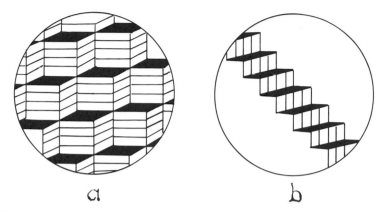

Fig. 12.5: Reversible cubes (a) and staircase (b). The black areas may appear to be the tops of the cubes (a) or staircase (b) or they may appear to be the bottoms. This reversibility of 'solid' forms exists due to the lack of perspective (depth) in the figures.

sharp and colour can be misleading. The psychologist Edgar Rubin (1915) stated that the visual world is regarded in terms of some figure(s) with the remainder as ground. The 'figure' is the form, the delineated and tangible aspect of the scene; while the ground is akin to background, it is poorly delineated, more amorphous than the figure and is seen to be behind the figure. However, line drawings exist in which a pair of shapes (either of which when taken alone would be seen as an object of some kind) share a common border-line. In such cases, figure-ground reversal occurs. Alternatively, one is relegated to mere background while the other dominates as subject; then this one fades away to become mere background in its place. Examples of visual reversal are given in Fig. 12.6. In these examples, perception fluctuates between two possibilities. This is noteworthy because it shows that perception is not simply determined by patterns at the retina; rather there must be some subtle process of interpretation even at this elementary level. Maltese crosses (Fig. 12.7) can also be taken as examples of figure-ground reversal, however, they also illustrate a partiality towards vertical orientation and the smallest area enclosed.

Paradoxes

All pictures are essentially paradoxes in that they are seen, in their own right, as flat objects of light, shade and colour; while at the same time they appear as quite different three-dimensional

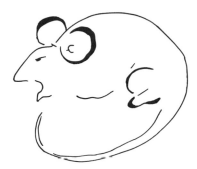

Fig. 12.6: Ambiguous figure. Rat and professor compete for recognition.
(From Bugelski & Alamprey, 1961)

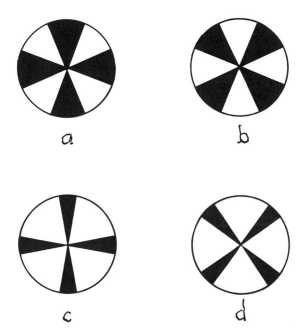

Fig. 12.7: Maltese crosses.
a, b -consist of equal alternate black and white segments. Yet
       the favoured figure is the black cross in (a) and the white
       cross in (b).   This shows that perception shows a
       partiality towards a vertical orientation.
c, d -the black cross is favoured as figure both in (c) and (d).
       This shows a partiality towards the smallest area
       enclosed.

objects in a different space. It is this double-reality of pictures which makes them unique as visual objects of perception. In addition to giving a three-dimensional appearance to a picture plane, artists can also do the reverse (make three-dimensional shapes appear flat) by employing deliberate misleading cues to distance; or even 'impossible' by paradoxes of depth. Thus it is possible to create a two-dimensional object (figure) for which a three-dimensional counterpart is highly unlikely. The prongs in Fig. 12.8a may not be puzzling at a glance, but close examination shows that they are 'impossible'. If the 'impossibility' is not perceived, this is probably due to fluctuation of alteration between the left and right sides of the figure, each of which by itself is quite possible, without a liaison between the two sides. Similarly, the top and bottom halves of Fig. 12.8b are both possible, but the figure as a whole is 'impossible'.

Some paradoxes can be resolved, others cannot. When a paradox is due to specifically given incompatible information it is not possible to resolve it without rejection of information. Paradoxes which can be resolved are those which are due to an inappropriate hypothesis adopted for reconciling the given elements. For example, in the 'impossible' triangle (Fig. 12.9), if the real three-dimensional shape (actually quite unlike the triangular image it gives from a critical position) is seen the paradox disappears. Thus, we see that this image is a special case, subsumed under the general perceptual hypothesis of the shape of the object which holds for any viewing position. The nearest we ever get to the truth is a hypothesis which, when accepted, gives no surprises in new situations.

Movement Distortion

Adaptation to one sensory channel but not to another which parallels it can lead to curious effects. Rotation of the spiral (Fig. 12.10) clockwise on a record-player turntable produces apparent expansion, while maintaining the same size. The after-effects, seen in the stationary phase, following rotation, are the reverse of those observed during rotation. To expand/shrink and yet to remain unchanged in size is impossible for any physical object; i.e. it is paradoxical. However, this is what is seen in this adaptation-illusion. This form of movement distortion is known as the 'waterfall effect' or the 'after-effect of seen motion'. Just why it occurs is unclear. Some theories suggest that it results from overload firing of the specialised cell circuits in the brain that respond to motion. Others feel that adaptation processes in the

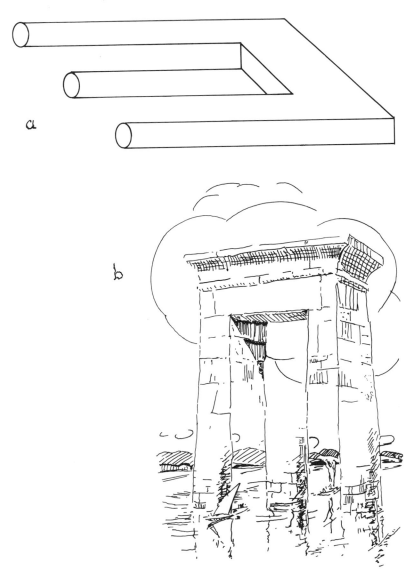

Fig. 12.8: (a) The 'impossible' prongs and (b) an interesting use of them.
(From Davidoff, 1975)

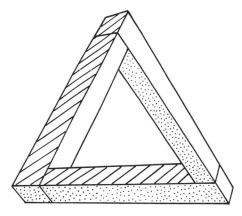

Fig. 12.9: 'Impossible' figures. This figure is seen as more than just mere patterns, however it is 'impossible' to see it as a possible object.
(After Penrose & Penrose, 1958)

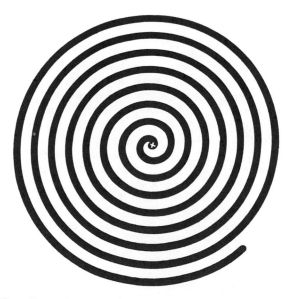

Fig. 12.10: Rotation of the spiral in a clockwise direction about its centre (white cross) produces an apparent expansion of the image; although it maintains the same size. After effects seen in the stationary phase following the rotation are the reverse seen during rotation.

retina are at least partially responsible. In any case a stationary reference within the visual field appears essential for the waterfall effect to occur. This is fortunate because otherwise we would suffer the waterfall effect at every sudden automobile stop!

Another form of motion distortion is the 'phi phenomenon'. It is the apparent movement experienced when the pages of a book are flipped, and is a phenomenon employed in motion pictures and television. It is also seen in commercial signs and marquees where single lights are flashed on and off in succession giving the impression of a moving image (e.g. an arrow). This visual phenomenon is strengthened by the persistence of vision which encourages the fusion of successive images and by one's tendency to group together into a meaningful whole stimuli that are similar in form and location.

In addition to the above, there are figures which can stimulate the eye so that it experiences movement. Grouping is one way by which the mind perceives figure-ground relationships from separate elements. In some, this strategy is rewarded by closure within a meaningful figure (Fig. 12.6), however this is not always possible. This is particularly true of overall patterns made up of many identical or nearly identical units; in this case the periodic structures tend to group and regroup themselves. Many perceptual organisations occur as the mind persists in trying to arrive at permanent closure. However, the effort is doomed as the visual stimulus lends itself to different possibilities. Thus, the figure appears to shift, and float, and shimmer; sometimes with violent illusory movement (Fig. 12.11). This property is employed skillfully by op(tical) artists, who abandon all hints of objects to produce designs which simulate motion. It is most likely that this sensation of movement is due to direct stimulation of the retinal movement detectors and the constant tremor of the eyes. At any rate, these effects seem to be caused by driving the neural systems beyond their normal functional limits and 'overloading' them. These effects are similar to the 'circuit faults' induced by drugs and fatigue.

Brightness and Colour Distortions

Adaptation to local regions of bright light gives well-known visual after-images (e.g. bright, dark or coloured). Transferring a gaze previously focussed on a bright, white light source, to a white wall or sheet of paper will result in a dark area (corresponding to the source of light) on a grey background. This has been explained

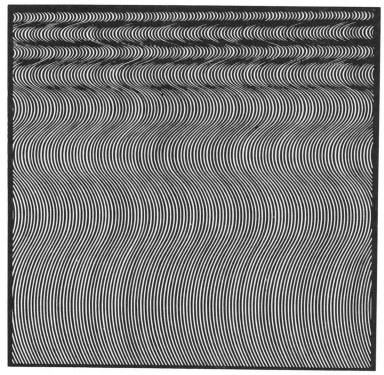

Fig. 12.11: Optical art. Eye movements play a part by stimulating the 'on-off' movement detectors of the retina and also by beating the repeated forms against displaced after-images, to give moiré patterns; but there may well be more to it.
(From Gregory, 1970)

on the basis of the reduced sensitivity of retinal photoreceptors. When gazing at a bright light source that part of the retina which is stimulated by the light transmits a strong signal to the brain; this part of the retina loses sensitivity. Shifting the gaze to an evenly lit surface results in a reduction of the signal from these retinal photoreceptors to the brain. Thus the relative reduction induces the 'dark-patch' which appears as the after-image of a bright light.

Colour effects are similar in origin. Colour is transmitted to the brain from the retina along (almost certainly) only three channels. There are three types of cone receptors, each sensitive to red, green or blue. White light activates all three colour channels, and the proportion from each 'means' white. Red light gives relatively more activity in the 'red' channel; green in the 'green' channel; and blue in the 'blue' channel. All colours are given by the proportional activity in the three colour channels. Now when one or more of the retinal colour systems has been adapted - to lose sensitivity by prolonged exposure to coloured light - the brain receives the same signal that it receives with light of the complementary colour of the adapting light. Thus the complementary colour is seen.

These after-image effects are known to be at least mainly due to retinal changes in the brain's projection areas with prolonged or violent stimulation of the eye. A more complicated effect, which is also probably retinal in origin, is the production of colour with flickering white light. If the disc (Fig. 12.12) is rotated it will gradually become coloured - the colours varying with the speed of rotation. The explanation is that the three retinal colour systems have (in electronic terminology) different time-constants. The rotating disc gives intermittent stimulation to the colour receptors. It is probable that the red-, green- and blue-sensitive receptors have somewhat different time-constants, so that repeated flashes of light build up different levels of activity in the three systems which is equivalent to a coloured light to the brain. The signals from the eye are identical and so the illusion of colour is compelling.

Summary

        Perception makes remarkably efficient use of strictly inadequate, thus ambiguous, information for selecting internally stored hypothesis of the current state of the external world. These are in terms of what kinds of objects are present and their sizes and appropriate positions in space. Object-recognition is further simplified by the fact that most familiar objects are largely redundant. For example, faces have two eyes, so only one needs to be seen; if there is an eye then there must be a nose; if a head then a body. Indeed it is the associated facts about familiar objects which make close-ups on film possible. But this method of reduction, applicable to objects, does not necessarily extend to setting sizes and distance scales. If for some reason, the size or distance scales are set incorrectly, related perceptual distortion of size or distance occurs. It is therefore necessary to inquire whether distortion illusions are related to the particular kinds of sensory information used for setting perceptual size and distance (constancy scaling).

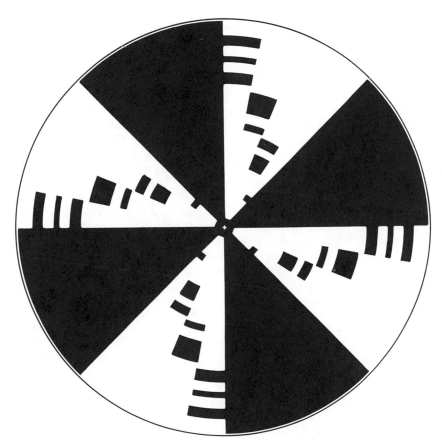

Fig. 12.12: Modified Benham's disc, although black and white will appear variously coloured if rotated. The colour signalling of the retina is upset by the time-spaced pulses of white and black. Any colour can be generated.
(From Gregory, 1970)

This could be the key to the problem of illusions, but there are other approaches. In visual distortions we have a system which is functioning, as expected, except in particular situations when viewing certain shapes. As all examples of the system (human observers) suffer similar errors, this error cannot be equivalent to a 'burned out component' of the neuro-circuit. Neurological abnormalities can also be ruled out as everyone appears to be similarly affected. There is, however, a possibility of circuit malfunction. The circuit may run into some kind of 'overload condition' as is apparent in the after-images of brightness and of colour, and the apparent movement perceived in op art.

A point worth mentioning when considering visual illusions is the relationship between cultures. This shows that perception is determined, at least partly, ecologically and the habitual exposures to pictures. Pictures are two-dimensional representations of what normally occur in three-dimensions; thus they can be interpreted in different ways depending on the 'experience' of the observer. To our eyes size denotes distance; but for cultures confined to limited surroundings (enclosures) there is practically no comprehension of size scaling. Thus a large distant object (which appears small) is interpreted as a small nearby object. Unfortunately several confounding factors (e.g. education, test sophistication, as well as physiological factors such as age and retinal pigmentation) are present in such studies. Nevertheless evidence from developmental and cross-cultural research supports a position of moderate empiricism. Findings from cross-cultural research (see Davidoff, 1975; Stewart, 1971) show small, but nonetheless real differences between experientially disparate groups in the way they perceive the visual world. Similarly, young organisms respond appropriately to certain ecologically important features of their environment without specific training or experience but show no really convincing demonstration of object perception or size and shape constancy.

This account of visual illusions is by no way complete or their explanation explicit, but if it has stimulated interest in the phenomena of visual illusions it has served its purpose.

13

EXTRAOCULAR PHOTORECEPTORS

Light is involved in several life-processes other than vision. Its innate importance may rest either in its energy content (e.g. photosynthesis) or in its function as a Zeitgeber, its energy content being secondary (e.g. vision). This latter aspect of light is also applicable to photomorphogenesis, photomovement, circadian rhythms and reproductive cycles. In these instances photoreception, as distinct from the simple absorption of light quanta, is involved. A characteristic of photoreception is that the energy required to process biological activities triggered by the reception of photons are completely out of proportion to the energy contained within the light stimulus itself. Conversely, carbon fixation in photosynthesis, cellular destruction by ultraviolet radiation, and to a lesser extent the degree of tanning of human skin are proportional to the number of quanta in the light which produces these effects. These processes are all mediated by photopigments. In photoreception, however, the pigments are located within specialised cells - photoreceptors.

An organism may possess multiple photopigments as well as multiple photoreceptors which may mediate different photic responses. However, because of our own subjective visual experience, we are surprised to learn that most highly developed organisms with complex image forming eyes also possess other less obvious photoreceptors which monitor crucially important aspects of the photic environment. At least some species, in each of the vertebrate classes, are known to depend on extraocular photoreception for the regulation of important aspects of their physiology and behaviour. This phenomenon has been convincingly identified in a great many studies involving birds, frogs, tadpoles, lizards, salamanders and fishes (see Adler, 1970). Extraocular photoreceptors include the pineal as well as undetermined and dermal photoreceptors.

Pineal

The pineal organ (epiphysis cerebri) develops as a sac-like evagination, or in some species as two diverticula, of the dorsal diencephalic roof. It is present in a wide number of vertebrates and its structure has been described in fishes, amphibians, reptiles, birds and mammals (Fig. 13.1). The pineal body and the pineal end organ (in amphibians), and their homologous structure, the parietal eye (in reptiles) are probably photoreceptive. Electrophysiological studies have come out strongly in support of the photoreceptive nature of the pineal in fishes, amphibians and reptiles. Structurally, specialised sensory cells have been found in vertebrate pineals. These cells range from highly ordered arrays of photoreceptors which resemble a simple retina; scattered, simple, outer segment-like organelles; and at the extreme end of the scale, the non-photoreceptive, secretory cells - pinealocytes - (Fig. 13.2). Photoreceptors in the pineal, as in the retina, are ciliary in origin and consist of a varying number of stacked lamellae which may be regular (cone-like), irregular (e.g. vesiculated), or dome-like (Fig. 13.3). Photopigments of the pineal photoreceptors are located on these stacked lamellae. The pineal eye of Xenopus laevis shows a maximal sensitivity to 520 nm which corresponds to the maximal sensitivity of their retinal rod photoreceptors. As the latter contain porphyropsin it is inferred that the pineal photoreceptors of this species also contain this pigment (Foster & Roberts, 1982). Although there are no known microspectrophotometric studies of pineal photoreceptors, if the above holds, then the pineal photoreceptors will contain similar photopigments to their counter-parts (i.e. rods) in the lateral eye. Thus one would expect to find porphyropsin in pineal photoreceptors of fresh water vertebrates and rhodopsin in pineal photoreceptors of marine and aerial/terresterial vertebrates.

The regression of pineal photoreceptors to rudimentary photoreceptors (pseudosensory cells); to sensory, secretory cells (pinealocytes) is thought to reflect the phylogenetic trend in vertebrates (Fig. 13.4). Thus, pineals of lower vertebrates, including lacertilian reptiles, contain well-developed photoreceptors; turtles, lizards and birds contain rudimentary photoreceptors; and mammals contain pinealocytes which are considered to have lost the ability of direct photoreception. However, exceptions to the latter exist. Rudimentary photoreceptor cells

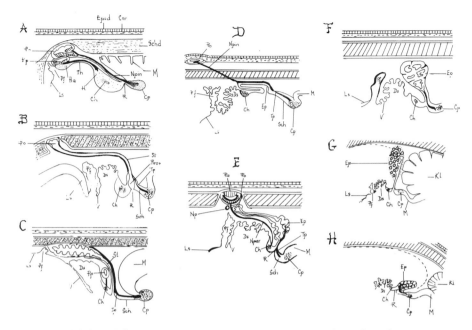

Fig. 13.1: Diagrammatic representation of the pineal organ and the parietal eye of various vertebrates.
A - Petromyzon; B- Elasmobranchii; C - Teleostei; D - Anura; E - Sauria; F - Ophidia; G - Aves; H - Mammalia.
Ch - commissura habenularis (H) superior; Cor - corium; Cp - commissura posterior; Ds - dorsal sac; Ep - epiphysis cerebri (corpus pineal, pineal body); Epid - epidermis; Ha - ganglion habenulae anterius; Kl cerebellum; Ls - lamina supraneuroporica; M - mesencephalon; Np - accessory parietal organ; Npar - nervus parietalis; Npin - nervus pinealis; Pa - parietal eye; Pf - paraphysis cerebri; Pp - parapineal organ; Prox - proximal part of the pineal organ; Po - pineal organ and frontal organ (pineal terminal vesicle); Sch - connecting piece; Schd - skull bone; St - stalk of the pineal organ; Th - tractus habenularis; Tp - tractus pinealis; V - velum transversum.
(After Oksche, 1965)

have been observed in the pineal of the adult noctule bat and the golden mole; while in the adult golden hamster even a cone-like structure was observed (see Nadakavukaren & Bucana, 1980).

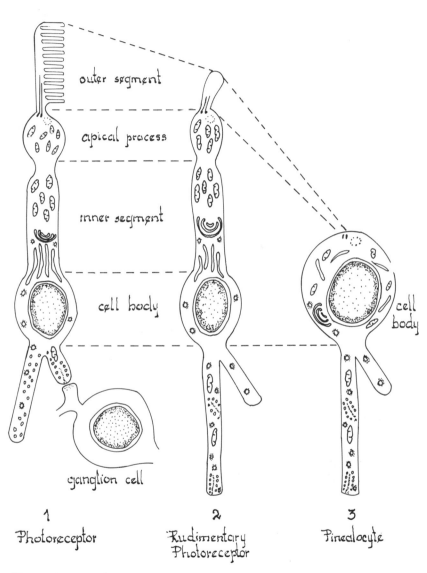

Fig. 13.2: Diagrammatic representation showing the transformation of pineal photoreceptors of vertebrates into pinealocytes.
(After Collin, 1969)

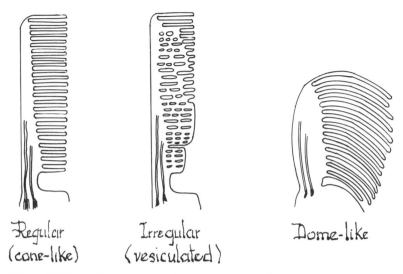

Regular
(cone-like)

Irregular
(vesiculated)

Dome-like

Fig. 13.3: Diagrammatic representation of various outer segment structures of pineal photoreceptors. (After Collin, 1969)

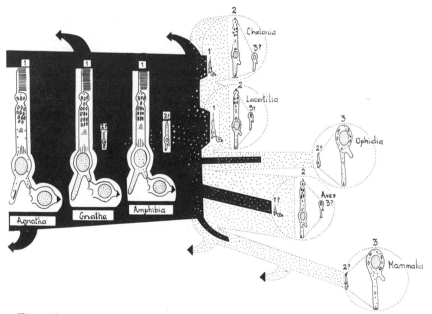

Fig. 13.4: Evolution of pineal sensory cells in vertebrates. 1 - photoreceptor; 2 - rudimentary photoreceptor; 3 - pinealocyte. (After Collin, 1969)

In lower vertebrates the pineal, as an extraocular photo-receptor, is hypothesised to relate environmental lighting to the behaviour and physiology of these animals. Thus the pineal has been shown to function as a dosimeter of solar radiation and as an indicator of day length (pike; Falcon & Meissl, 1981); a regulator of orientation behaviour and locomotor activity patterns (Adler, 1970; Taylor & Adler, 1978); and as a detector of the e-vector direction of environmental polarised light (Ambystoma tigrinum; Hartwig & Korf, 1978).

Photoreceptive capabilities of the pineal and its associated responses can be determined through experimentation with normal, blinded, pinealectomised and pinealectomised-blinded individuals in conjunction with histochemical, immunocytochemical, biochemical, ultrastructural and electrophysiological techniques. These studies demonstrated that pineal photoreceptors, like retinal photo-receptors, usually respond to light stimulus by an inhibition of spontaneous neuronal activity (achromatic response). Light causes hyperpolarisation of the photoreceptor membrane and inhibits the spontaneous discharge of ganglion cells. Pineal photoreceptors also contain synaptic ribbons which increase in number and size during the night and under continuous darkness, whereas they decrease during the day and under continuous light (Omura & Ali, 1981). In addition, the pineal also contains indoles (e.g. 5-hydroxytryptophan; 5-hydroxytryptamine (serotonin); and melatonin) and associated enzymes (e.g. hydroxyindole-O-methyl transferase, HIOMT) which have been shown to fluctuate with the daily light/dark cycles (Fig. 13.5). The levels of these neurosecretory products are thought to be related to the type of dense-cored vesicles present within the pineal cells (see Omura & Ali, 1981). The rhythmic production and release of these compounds (predominantly serotonin and melatonin) may modulate reproductive cycles among other physiol-ogical processes.

Brain and Dermal Photoreceptors

The persistence of photoresponses in blinded-pinealectomised individuals (e.g. eel, minnows, sparrow, pigeon) indicate that there are other extraretinal photoreceptors besides the pineal (Fig. 13.6). Very much less is known about these photoreceptors which may be deep-seated encephalic photoreceptors or dermal photoreceptors located in regions other than the head.

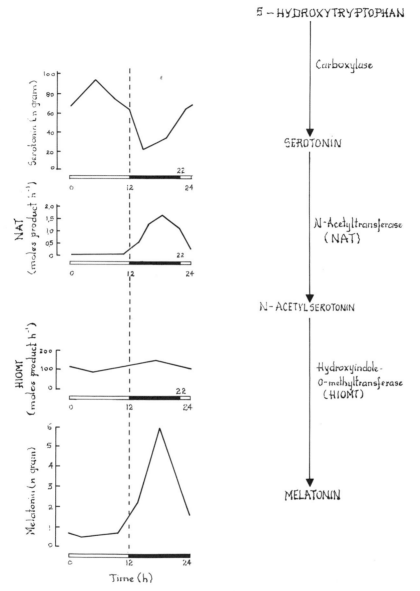

Fig. 13.5: Diagrammatic representation of biological rhythms in the adult rat pineal gland. All light-dark cycles were LD - 14:10 except for the melatonin data which was LD - 12:12. (From Binkley, 1983)

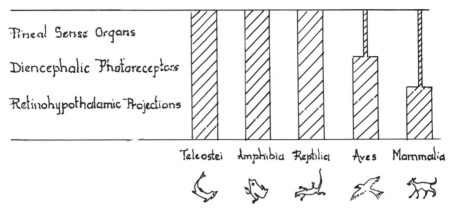

Fig. 13.6: Comparative survey indicating the presence of pineal sense organs (1); diencephalic photoreceptors (2); and retinohypothalamic projections (3) in the vertebrate phylum. Hatched columns - presence of photosensory system indicated on the left side of the diagram. Hatched line - photosensory capacity not shown in threshold experiments. Only limited numbers of species have been investigated. (From Hartwig, 1982)

Encephalic Photoreceptors

Vertebrates, with the apparent exception of mammals, possess encephalic photoreceptive areas within the vicinity of the wall of the third ventricle. Visible radiation can penetrate into all parts of the body, including the hypothalamus (Wurtman, 1975). Recordings of spectral transmission (400 - 750 nm) showed that visible radiation of longer wavelengths (700 - 750 nm) penetrated more efficiently than the shorter wavelengths (400 - 450 nm). Thus, encephalic photoreceptors in large vertebrates will be more sensitive to longer wavelengths. Microspectrophotometric measurements showed that the ependymal area of the anterio-dorsal hypothalamus of minnows and goldfish (body lengths 2 - 4 cm) and tadpoles of Rana temporaria contained a photolabile compound with an ill-defined absorption maximum between 560 - 580 nm. However, regularly laminated structures (representing outer segments) have not been observed in the areas containing this photolabile compound. Thus its integrity as a photopigment is questionable. In addition, this photopigment detectable in small minnows (body length 2 - 4 cm) is no longer detectable in larger individuals (body length 10 -14 cm). On the other hand, house sparrows while exhibiting encephalic photoreception show no evidence of photolabile compounds in the diencephalon (Menaker, 1977).

At the ultrastructural level, the area of the teleost brain containing a photolabile compound also contains cells with bulbous cilia of the sensory type (9 + 0) which resembles the early developmental stages of retinal and pineal photoreceptor outer segments or cerebrospinal fluid containing neurones. However, structures rich in mitochondria (corresponding to the ellipsoids of retinal photoreceptors) have not been found in association with the bulbous cilia.

Encephalic photoreceptors detect luminous flux reaching the diencephalon, without analysing the spatial intensity differences. This function can be accomplished by unlamellated outer segments distributed over a large surface. The luminous flux is compared with the expected level indicated by the phase angle of the "biological clock", which can be fulfilled by membrane bound photopigments distributed over a large surface. Thus, it is uncertain if all the neurones lining the third ventricle have photosensory functions or even if this function can be attributed to specialised cells. It should be remembered that only a limited, though constant, number of photosensory cells is required to record the penetration of light into the diencephalon. Thus, with increasing brain size, these cells may be scattered over a large area.

The functions of the encephalic photoreceptors are varied. In eels, these photoreceptors are responsible for the synchronisation of circadian motor activity with the external photoperiod, and for the control of photonegative behaviour (van Veen et al., 1976). In birds, encephalic photoreceptors apparently control gonadal growth (Menaker, 1971; Yokoyama et al., 1978).

Dermal Photoreceptors

In some species of vertebrates, occlusion of the whole head from light still results in responsiveness to photostimulation. This indicates that the response is not directly mediated by either the retina, pineal or encephalic photoreceptors; rather some form of dermal sensitivity would best account for the photoresponse. Dermal photic response is defined as that response which is mediated by receptors located within the dermis. These receptors can be differentiated from heat receptors by virtue of their responsiveness to visible radiation (400 - 700 nm) and morphological attributes. In addition, they are distinct in that they do not exist as part of or in direct association with the brain.

In three of the species investigated (pigeon, chicken, ring-dove) only pigeons showed non-visual dermal light sensitivity (Heaton & Harth, 1974). The dermal light sensitivity of pigeons is characterised by an overt response of short latency to the onset of low intensity. The most intriguing possible significance of non-visual responsiveness to light in pigeons is the role it may play in homing. Even under conditions of rather severe visual impairment many birds retain their homing ability thereby indicating that the visual system may not be involved in this response at all.

Even less is known about dermal photoreceptors. Practically nothing is known about their location, structure or physiology. When considering structure, function and location of brain and dermal photoreceptors other factors such as the effects of light on enzymes (photosensitivity, oscillatory fluctuations of activities, relationship to photochromic compounds such as carotenoids and haemoproteins) should also be considered.

Summary

In summary, it can be seen that there is no complete case of extraocular photoreception. On the one hand there is no clear picture of the function of the extraocular photoreceptors which have been identified and their physiology studied (pineal). While on the other, the functions are known (e.g. entrainment) but the precise localisation, structure and physiology of the photoreceptors are unknown (encephalic and dermal photoreceptors).

The presence of extraocular photoreception in vertebrates with well developed visual capabilities raises the interesting question of the selective advantage of partioning photoreceptivity into retinal and extraretinal photoreception. It is quite likely that there is some adaptive significance. In some cases extraocular photosensitivity is limited to early post-natal life (new-born rat; Zweig et al., 1966), or the presence of photolabile compounds in encephalic photoreceptors of small-sized specimens (minnows; Hartwig, 1975). These findings raise a whole series of questions concerning the developmental events which lead to the loss of these extraocular photoreceptors. Thus the field of extraocular photoreception is still wide open to research. The identity, function and physiological characteristics of each of the different types of extraocular photoreceptors in particular await further study.

REFERENCES

Abramov I (1968) Further analysis of the responses of LGN cells. J Opt Soc Am 58: 574

Adler KK (1970) The role of extraocular photoreceptors in amphibian rhythms and orientation: A review. J Herpetol 4: 99

Ali MA (1971) Les réponses rétinomotrices: Caractères et mécanismes. Vision Res 11: 1225

Ali MA (1975) Retinomotor responses. In: Ali MA (ed), Vision in fishes. Plenum, New York, p 313

Ali MA (1981) Adaptations rétiniennes aux habitats. Rev Can Biol 40: 3

Ali MA, Anctil M (1977) Retinal structure and function in the walleye (Stizostedion vitreum) and sauger (S. canadense). J Fish Res Bd Can 34: 1467

Ali MA, Crouzy R (1968) Action spectrum and quantal thresholds of retinomotor responses in the brook trout, Salvelinus fontinalis, (Mitchill). Z verg Physiol 59: 86

Ali MA, Harosi FI, Wagner HJ (1978) Photoreceptors and visual pigments in a cichlid fish Nannacara anomala. Sen Proc 2: 130

Ali MA, Klyne MA (1983) Phylogeny and functional morphology of of the vertebrate retina. In: Functional morphology in vertebrates. International symposium on vertebrate morphology, Giessen, August 22-26, 1983

Ali MA, Wagner HJ (1980) Vision in charrs: Review and perspectives. In: Balon EK (ed), Charrs: Salmonid fishes of the genus Salvelinus. Dr. W Junk, The Hague, p 391

Allen DM, Loew ER, McFarland WN (1982) Seasonal change in the amount of visual pigment in the retinae of fish. Can J Zool 6: 281

241

Anctil M, Ali MA, Couillard P (1980) Cone myoid elongation and rod myoid contraction are inhibited by colchicine in the trout retina. Experientia 36: 574

Armington JC (1955) Amplitude of response and relative sensitivity of the human electroretinogram. J Opt Soc Am 45: 1058

Armington JC (1974) The electroretinogram. Academic Press, New York, pp 478

Armington JC, Crampton GH (1958) Comparison of spectral sensitivity at the eye and the optic tectum of the chicken. Am J Ophthalmol 46: 72

Athanassious R (1983) La transduction visuelle dans la rétine de la truite mouchetée (Salvelinus fontinalis, Mitchill): Approche cytochimique. Ph D Thesis. Université de Montréal, Montréal, Canada

Athanassious R, Klyne MA, Ali MA (1984) Ultracytochemical evidence of calcium in the visual process. Mikroskopie 41: 4

Bader CR, MacLeish PR, Schwartz EA (1979) A voltage-clamp study of the light response in solitary rods of the tiger salamander. J Physiol 296: 1

Barlow HB (1972) Dark and light adaptation. In: Jameson D, Hurvich LM (eds), Handbook of sensory physiology, vol VII/4. Springer-Verlag, New York, Heidelberg, p 1

Beacher WJ (1952) The role of vision in alighting of birds. Science 115: 607

Berger ER (1966) On the mitochondrial origin of oil drops in the retinal double cone inner segments. J Ultrastruct Res 14: 143

Binkley SA (1983) Circadian rhythms of pineal function in rats. Endocrine Rev 4: 255

Birukow G (1952) Vergleichende Unterschungen über das Helligkeitsund Farbensehen bei Amphibien. Z verg Physiol 32: 348

Birukow G, Knoll M (1952) Tages und Dammerungssehen von Froschlarven nach Aufzucht in verschiedenen Lichtbedingungen. Naturwiss 21: 494

Bitensky MW, Wheeler GL, Yamazaki A, Rasenick MM, Stein PJ (1981) Cyclic nucleotide metabolism in vertebrate photoreceptors: A remarkable analogy and an unraveling enigma. Curr Top Memb Transp 15: 237

Blaurock AE, Wilkins MH (1969) Structure of frog photoreceptor membranes. Nature 223(5209): 909

Blaxter HJS, Jones MP (1967) The development of the retina and retinomotor responses in the herring. J Mar Biol Assoc UK 47: 677

Blaxter JHS, Staines M (1970) Pure-cone retinae and retinomotor responses in larval teleosts. J Mar Biol Assoc UK 50: 449

Bloomer CM (1976) Principles of visual perception. Van-Nostrand
    Reinhold Co, New York, pp 148

Bonaventure N (1961) La vision des couleurs chez le chat. Rev
    Psychol Franç 6: 1

Bowmaker JK (1980) Colour vision in birds and the role of oil
    droplets. Trends Neurosci August 1980: 196

Bowmaker JK, Dartnall HJA, Lythgoe JN, Mollon JD (1978) The
    visual pigments of rods and cones in the rhesus monkey. J
    Physiol 274: 329

Bowmaker JK, Martin GR (1978) Visual pigment and colour vision
    in a nocturnal bird, Strix aluco (Tawny owl). Vision Res 18:
    1125

Boycott BB, Dowling JE (1969) Organization of the primate retina:
    Light microscopy. Phil Trans R Soc Lond 255B: 14

Boynton RM, Gordon J (1965) Bezold-Brücke hue shift measured by
    colour naming techniques. J Opt Soc Am 55: 78

Bridges CDB (1967) Spectroscopic properties of porphyropsins.
    Vision Res 7: 349

Brin KP, Ripps H (1977) Rhodopsin photoproducts and rod
    sensitivity in the skate retina. J Gen Physiol 69: 97

Bugelski BR, Alamprey DA (1961) The role of frequency in
    developing perceptual sets. Can J Psychol 15: 205

Burns BD, Pritchard R (1971) Geometrical illusions and the
    response of neurons in the cat's visual cortex to angle
    patterns. J Physiol 213: 599

Burnside B (1978) Thin (actin) and thick (myosin-like) filaments in
    cone contraction in the teleost retina. J Cell Biol 78: 227

Caspersson TO (1940) Methods for the determination of the
    absorption spectra of cell structures. J R Microsc Soc 60: 8

Chiang C (1968) A new theory to explain geometrical illusions
    produced by crossing lines. Perception Psychophys 3: 174

Chievitz JH (1889) Unterschungen über die Area centralis retinae.
    Arch Anat Physiol Anat abt Suppl 139

Clarke GL (1939) The utilization of solar energy by aquatic
    organisms. Am Assoc Adv Sci 10: 27

Cohen AI (1972) Rods and cones. In: Fuortes MGF (ed), Handbook
    of sensory physiology, vol VII/2. Spginger-Verlag, New York,
    Heidelberg, p 63

Cohen AI, Hall IA, Ferrendelli JA (1978) Calcium and cyclic
    nucleotide regulation in incubated mouse retinas. J Gen
    Physiol 71: 595

Collin JP (1969) Contributions à l'étude de l'organe pinéal. De
    l'épiphyse sensorielle à la glande pinéale: Modalités de
    transformation et implications fonctionnelles. Annales de la
    station biologique de Besse-en-Chaudesse, Supp 1

Colvin SS, Burford CC (1909) The colour perception of three dogs, a cat and a squirrel. Psychol Monogr 11: 1

Couillard P (1975) Approaches to the study of contractility in the rods and cones. In: Ali MA (ed), Vision in fishes: New approaches in research. Plenum, New York, p 357

Crescitelli F (1967) Extraction of visual pigments with certain alkyl phenoxy polyethoxy ethanol surface-active compounds. Vision Res 7: 685

Crescitelli F (1972) The visual cells and visual pigments of the vertebrate eye. In: Dartnall HJA (ed), Handbook of sensory physiology, vol VII/1. Springer-Verlag, New York, Heidelberg, p 245

Dartnall HJA (1953) The interpretation of spectral sensitive curves. Br Med Bull 9: 24

Dartnall HJA (1957) The visual pigments. Methuen & Co Ltd, London, pp 216

Dartnall HJA (1961) Visual pigments before and after extraction from visual cells. Proc R Soc Lond 154B: 250

Dartnall HJA, Lythgoe JN (1965) The spectral clustering of pigments. Vision Res 5: 81

Davidoff JB (1975) Differences in visual perception. The individual eye. Academic Press, New York, pp 231

Davson H (ed) (1977) The eye, vol 2: The photobiology of vision. Academic Press, New York, pp 689

Day RH (1972) Visual spatial illusions: A general explanation. Science 175: 1335

Denison RH (1956) A review of the habitat of the earliest vertebrates. Fieldiana: Geology 11: 359

Denton EJ (1954) On the orientation of molecules in the visual rods of Salamandra maculosa. J Physiol 124: 17

Denton EJ (1956) Recherches sur l'absorption de la lumière par le cristallin des poissons. Bull Inst Oceanogr, Monaco 1071: 1

Denton EJ, Gilpin-Brown JB, Wright PG (1970) On the 'filter' in the photophores of mesopelagic fish and on a fish emitting red light and especially sensitive to red light. J Physiol Lond 208: 72

Denton EJ, Wyllie JH (1955) Study of the photosensitive pigments in the pink and green rods of the frog. J Physiol 127: 81

DeValois DL (1965) Analysis and coding of color vision in the primate visual system. Cold Spring Harb Symp Quant Biol 30: 567

DeValois RL (1973) Central mechanisms of color vision. In: Jung R (ed), Handbook of sensory physiology, vol VII/3. Springer-Verlag, New York, Heidelberg, p 209

DeValois RL, Abramov I, Jacobs GH (1966) Analysis of response patterns of LGN cells. J Opt Soc Am 56: 966

DeValois RL, Marrocco RT (1971) Single cell analysis of saturation discrimination in the macaque. Vision Res 13: 701

Dobrowolski JA, Johnson BK, Tansley K (1955)   The spectral absorption of the photopigment of Xenopus laevis measured in single rods. J Physiol 130: 533

Dodt E (1954)   Ergebnisse der Flimmer-Elektroretinographie. Experientia 10: 330

Dodt E, Walther JB (1959)   Über die spektrale Empfindlighkeit und die Schwelle von Gecko-Augen. Pflüger's Arch 268: 204

Donner KO, Reuter T (1968)   Visual adaptation of rhodopsin rods in the frog's retina. J Physiol 199: 59

Dowling JE, Boycott BB (1966) Organization of the primate retina: Electron microscopy. Proc R Soc Lond 166B: 80

Duijm M (1959) On the position of a ribbon-like central area in the eyes of some birds. Arch Neerl Zool 13 (Supp 1): 128

du Pont YS, de Groot PJ (1976) A schematic dioptric apparatus for the frog's eye (Rana esculenta). Vision Res 16: 803

Eakin RM (1962) Lines of evolution of photoreceptors. J Gen Physiol 46: 357A

Ebbesson SOE (1972) A proposal for a common nomenclature for some optic nuclei in vertebrates and the evidence for a common origin of two such cell groups. Brain Behav Evol 6: 75

Ebrey TG, Hoing B (1975)   Molecular aspects of photoreceptor function. Quant Rev Biophys 8: 129

Falcon J, Meissl H (1981) The photosensory function of the pineal organ of the pike (Esox lucius L.):   Correlation between structure and function. J Comp Physiol 144: 127

Farber DB (1981) Cyclic AMP enrichment in retinal cones. Curr Top Memb Transp 15: 231

Fein A, Szuts EZ (1982) Photoreceptors: Their role in vision. Cambridge University Press, Cambridge, London, New York, pp 212

Ferrero E, Anctil M, Ali, MA (1979) Ultrastructural correlates of retinomotor responses in inner segments of vertebrate photo-receptors. Rev Can Biol 38: 249

Foster RG, Roberts A (1982) The pineal eye in Xenopus laevis embryos and larvae. A photoreceptor with a direct excitatory effect on behaviour. J Comp Physiol 145A: 413

Fung BKK, Hubbel WL (1978)   Organization of rhodopsin in photoreceptor membranes. II. Transmembrane organization of bovine rhodopsin: Evidence from proteolysis and lacto-peroxidase-catalyzed iodination of native and reconstituted membranes. Biochem 17: 4403

Ganz L (1966) Is the figural after effect an after effect? Psychol Bull 58: 403

Gardner E (1975)   The special senses and their pathways. In:

Fundamentals of neurology: A psychophysiological approach. WB Saunders Co, Philadelphia, London, Toronto, Sixth Edition, pp 460

Gibson KS, Tyndall EPT (1923-24) The visibility of radient energy. Bull Nat Bur Standards 19: 131

Gordis C, Urban PF, Mandel P (1977) The effect of flash illumination on the endogenous cyclic GMP content of isolated frog retina. Exp Eye Res 24: 171

Govardovskii VI, Berman AL (1981) Light-induced changes of cyclic GMP content in frog retinal rod outer segments measured with rapid freezing and microdissection. Biophys Struct Mech 7: 125

Grabowski SR, Pak WL (1975) Intracellular recordings of rod responses during dark-adaptation. J Physiol 247: 363

Graeber RC, Ebbesson SOE (1972) Visual discrimination in learning in normal and tectal-ablated nurse sharks (Ginglymostoma cirratum). Comp Biochem Physiol 42A: 131

Graeber RC, Ebbesson SOE, Jane JA (1973) Visual discrimination in sharks without optic tectum. Science 180: 413

Gramoni R, Ali MA (1970) L'électrorétinogramme et sa fréquence de fusion chez Amia calva (Linné). Rev Can Biol 29: 353

Granit R (1947) Sensory mechanisms of the retina. Oxford Univ Press, London, New York, Toronto, pp 412

Granit R, Munsterhjelm A (1937) The electrical responses of dark adapted frog's eyes to monochromatic stimuli. J Physiol 88: 436

Granit R, Wrede CM (1937) The electrical responses of light adapted frog's eyes to monochromatic stimuli. J Physiol 89: 239

Gregory RL (1970) The intelligent eye. McGraw-Hill Book Co, New York, pp 191

Grzimek B (1952) Versuche über das Farbensehen von Pflanzenessern. I. Das farbige Sehen von Pferde. Z Tierpsychol 9: 23

Gundlach RH, Chard RD, Skahen JR (1945) The mechanism of accommodation in pigeons. J Comp Psychol 38: 27

Hagins WA, Yoshikami S (1974) A role for Ca^{++} in excitation of retinal rods and cones. Exp Eye Res 18: 299

Hanyu I, Ali, MA (1964) Electroretinogram and its flicker fusion frequency at different temperatures in light-adapted salmon (Salmo salar). J Cell Comp Physiol 63: 309

Hargrave PA, Fong SL, McDowell JH, Mas MT, Curtis DR (1980) The partial primary structure of bovine rhodopsin and its topography in the retinal rod cell disc membrane. Neurochem Int 1: 231

Harosi, FI (1981) Microspectrophotometry and optical phenomena:

Birefringence, dichroism and anomalous dispersion. In: Enoch JM, Tobey FL (eds), Vertebrate photoreceptor optics, Springer series in optical sciences, vol 23. Springer-Verlag, New York, Heidelberg, p 337

Harosi F (1982) Recent results from single-cell microspectrophotometry: Cone pigments in frog, fish and monkey. Color Res Appn 7: 135

Harosi FI, Hashimoto Y (1983) Ultraviolet visual pigment in a vertebrate: A tetrachromatic cone system in the dace. Science 222: 1021

Hartwig HG (1975) Neurobiologische Studien an photoneuroendokrinen Systemen. Habilitationsschrift in Bereich Humanmedzin der Justus Liebig-Universität Giessen

Hartwig HG, Korf HW (1978) The epiphysis cerebri of poikilothermic vertebrates: A photosensitive neuroendocrine circumventricular organ. Scan Elect Microsc 2: 163

Hartwig HG (1982) Comparative aspects of retinal and extraretinal photosensory input channels in entraining endogeneous rhythms. In: Ascholl J, Dann S, Groos G (eds), Vertebrate circadian rhythms. Springer-Verlag, Berlin, Heidelberg, p 26

Heaton MB, Harth MS (1974) Non-visual light responsiveness in the pigeon: Developmental and comparative considerations. J Exp Zool 188: 251

Hecht S (1928) The relation between visual acuity and illumination. J Gen Physiol 11: 255

Helmholtz H (1896) Handbuch der Physiologischen Optik. Hamburg & Leipzig, Second Edition

Hering E (1878) Zur Lehre vom Lichtsinne. Karl Gerolds Sohn, Wien

Hermann G (1958) Beiträge sur Physiologie des Rattenauges. Z Tierpsychol 15: 462

Hess C von (1912) Vergleichende Physiologie des Gesichtsinnes. Handbuch der vergleichende Physiologie. Fischer, Jena 4: 1

Hood C, Rushton WAK (1971) The Florida retinal densitometer. J Physiol 217: 213

Howland HC (1983) Optics and accommodation in owls and flying foxes. In: Huber F, Markl H (eds), Neuroethology and behavioral physiology. Springer-Verlag, Berlin, Heidelberg, p 153

Hubbard R (1958) The thermal stability of rhodopsin. J Gen Physiol 42: 259

Hubbell WL (1975) Characterization of rhodopsin in synthetic systems. Acc Chem Res 8: 85

Hubbell WL, Bownds MD (1979) Visual transduction in vertebrate photoreceptors. Ann Rev Neurosci 2: 17

Jacobs GH, Gaylord HA (1967) Effects of chromatic adaptation on color naming. Vision Res 7: 645

Jane JA, Levey N, Carlson NJ (1972) Tectal and cortical function in vision. Exp Neurol 35: 61

Jerlov NG (1970) Light: General introduction. In: Kinne O (ed), Marine ecology. A comprehensive integrated treatise on life in oceans and coastal waters. Vol 1, Environmental factors. Wiley-Interscience, New York, p 95

Kaneko A (1970) Physiological and morphological identification of horizontal, bipolar and amacrine cells in goldfish retina. J Physiol 207: 623

Kaupp UB, Schnetkamp PPM (1982) Calcium metabolism in vertebrate photoreceptors. Cell Calcium 3: 83

Kilbride P (1980) Calcium effects on frog retinal cGMP levels and their light-initiated rate of decay. J Gen Physiol 75: 457

Kilbride P, Ebrey TG (1979) Light-initiated changes of cyclic guanosine monophosphate levels in the frog retina measured with quick-freezing techniques. J Gen Physiol 74: 415

Kirschfeld K (1974) The absolute sensitivity of lens and compound eyes. Z Naturforsch 29C: 592

Knowles A, Dartnall HJA (1977) The photobiology of vision. In: Davson H (ed), The eye, vol 2B. Academic Press, New York, pp 689

Kolb H (1970) Organization of the outer plexiform layer of the primate retina: Electron microscopy of Golgi-impregnated cells. Phil Trans R Soc Lond 258B: 261

Kolb H, Boycott BB, Dowling JE (1969) A second type of midget bipolar cell in the primate retina. Phil Trans R Soc Lond 255B: 177

Kohlrausch A (1931) Tagersehen, Dämmerschen, Adaptation. Handbuch der Normalen und Pathologischen Physiologie 12: 1499

Kolmer W (1924) Über das Auge des Eisvogels (Alcedo attis attis). Pflüger's Arch 204: 266

König A (1894) Über den menschlichen Sehpurpur und seine Bedeutung für das Sehen. Sitzungsberichte Akademie der Wissenschaften 27: 577

Kries J von (1896) Über die Funktion der Netzhautstäbchen. Z Psychol 9: 81

Kropf A (1982) A new detergent for the study of visual pigments. Vision Res 22: 495

Kühne W (1878) On the photochemistry of the retina and on visual purple. Macmillan, London

Le Grand Y (1957) Light, colour and vision. Wiley, New York (English translation of Optique physiologique, lumière et couleurs, vol II. Revue d'optique, Paris, 1948)

Levine JS, MacNichol EF (1979) Visual pigments in teleost fishes:

Effects of habitat, microhabitat and behavior on visual system evolution. Sensory Proc 3: 95

Levine JS, MacNichol EF (1982) Color vision in fishes. Sci Am 246: 140

Lewin R (1985) Unexpected progress in photoreception. Science 227: 500

Liebman PA (1978) Rod disk calcium movement and transduction: A poorly illuminated story. Ann NY Acad Sci 307: 642

Liebman PA, Carroll S, Laties A (1969) Spectral sensitivity of retinal screening pigment migration in the frog. Vision Res 9: 377

Linsdale JM (1946) The California ground squirrel. University California Press

Lipetz LE (1962) A neural mechanism of the Purkinje shift. Am J Optometry Arch Am Acad Optometry Monograph No. 299

Lipton SA, Dowling JE (1981) The relation between Ca^{++} and cyclic GMP in rod photoreceptors. Curr Top Memb Transp 15: 381

Locket NA (1971) Retinal structure in Platytroctes apus a deep-sea fish with a pure rod fovea. J Mar Biol Assoc UK 51: 79

Lockie JD (1952) A comparison of some aspects of the retinae of the Manx shearwater, fulmar petrel and house sparrow. Quart J Microsc Sci 93: 347

Loew ER, Dartnall HJA (1976) Vitamin A_1/A_2-based visual pigment mixtures in cones of the rudd. Vision Res 16: 891

Lythgoe JN (1972) The adaptation of visual pigments to the photic environment. In: Dartnall HJA (ed), Handbook of sensory physiology, vol VII/1. Springer-Verlag, New York, p 566

Lythgoe JN (1979) The ecology of vision. Oxford University Press, Oxford, pp 244

MacNichol EF (1978) A photon-counting microspectrophotometer for the study of single vertebrate photoreceptor cells. In: Cool SJ, Smith EL (eds), Frontiers in visual science. Springer, New York, Heidelberg, p 194

MacNichol EF, Feinberg R, Harosi FI (1973) Colour discrimination processes in the retina. Proc 2nd Cong Int Colour Assoc Colour 73, p 191

MacNichol EF, Svaetichin G (1958) Electric responses from the isolated retinas of fishes. Am J Ophthalmol 46(Part II): 26

Mariani AP (1982) Biplexiform cells: Ganglion cells of the primate retina that contact photoreceptors. Science 216: 1134

Mariani AP, Leure-duPree AE (1978) Photoreceptors and oil droplet colors in the red area of the pigeon retina. J Comp Neurol 182: 821

Marshall J, Mellerio J, Palmer DA (1973) A schematic eye for the pigeon. Vision Res 13: 2449

Marshall NB (1971) Explorations in the life of fishes. Harvard University Press, Cambridge, Mass

Martin GR (1977) Absolute visual threshold and scotopic spectral sensitivity in the tawny owl, Strix aluco. Nature 268: 636

Mas MT, Wang JK, Hargrave PA (1980) Topography of rhodopsin in rod outer segment disk membranes; Photochemical labeling with N-(4-azido-2-nitrophenyl)-2-aminoethanesulfonate. Biochem 19: 684

McEwen WK (1959) The yellow pigment of human lenses. Am J Ophthalmol 47 (No. 5, pt II): 144

Menaker M (1971) Rhythms, reproduction, and photoreception. Biol Reprod 4: 295

Menaker M (1977) Extraretinal photoreception. In: Smith KC (ed), The science of photobiology. Plenum Press, New York, p 227

Menezes NA, Wagner HJ, Ali MA (1981) Retinal adaptations in fishes from a flood plain environment in the central Amazon basin. Rev Can Biol 40: 111

Meyer DB, Cooper TG, Gernez C (1965) Retinal oil droplets. In: Rohen JW (ed), The structure of the eye II, Symposium. Schattauer-Verlag, Stuttgart, p 521

Middleton WEK (1952) Vision through the atmosphere. Toronto University Press, Toronto

Miller WH (ed) (1981) Current topics in membranes and transport. Vol 15, Molecular mechanisms of photoreceptor transduction. Academic Press, New York, pp 452

Motokawa K (1970) Physiology of color and pattern vision. Igaku Shoin Ltd, Tokyo, pp 283

Munk O (1977) The visual cells and retinal tapetum of the foveate deep-sea fish Scopelasaurus lepidus (Teleostei). Zoomorphol 87: 21

Muntz WRA (1972) Inert absorbing and reflecting pigments. In: Dartnall HJA (ed), Handbook of sensory physiology, vol VII/1. Springer-Verlag, Berlin, p 529

Muntz WRA (1975) The visual consequences of yellow filtering pigments in the eyes of fishes occupying different habitats. In: Evans GC, Bainbridge R, Rackham O (eds), Light as an ecological factor II. Blackwell Sci Publ, Oxford, London, p 271

Munz FW, McFarland WN (1975) Part I. Presumptive cone pigments extracted from tropical marine fishes. Vision Res 15: 1045

Munz FW, McFarland WN (1977) Evolutionary adaptations of fishes to the photic environment. In: Crescitelli E (ed), Handbook of sensory physiology, vol VII/5. Springer-Verlag, Berlin, p 193

Munz FW, Schwanzara SA (1967) A nomogram for retinene$_2$-based visual pigments. Vision Res 7: 111

Nadakavukaren MJ, Bucana CD (1980) Cone-like structure in the pineal gland of the hamster. J Submicrosc Cytol 12: 691

Necker LA (1832) Observations on some remarkable phenomena seen in Switerzerland and an optical phenomenon which occurs on viewing a crystal or geometrical solid. Phil Mag 1: 329

Nicol JAC (1961) The tapetum in Scyliorhinus canicula. J Mar Biol Assoc UK 41: 271

O'Day WT, Fernandez HR (1974) Aristostomias scintillans (Malacoateidae): A deep-sea fish with visual pigments apparently adapted to its own bioluminescence. Vision Res 14: 545

O'Connor P, Burnside B (1981) Actin dependent cell elongation in teleost retinal rods: Requirement for actin filament assembly. J Cell Biol 89: 517

Oksche A (1965) Survey of the development and comparative morphology of the pineal organ. Prog Brain Res 10: 3

Omura Y, Ali MA (1981) Ultrastructure of the pineal organ of the killifish, Fundulus heteroclitus, with special reference to the secretory functions. Cell Tissue Res 219: 355

Padgham CA, Saunders JE (1975) The perception of light and colour. Academic Press, New York, pp 192

Pankhurst NW (1984) Retinal development in larval and juvenile European eel, Anguilla anguilla L. Can J Zool 62: 335

Parthe V (1972) Horizontal, bipolar and oligopolar cells in the teleost retina. Vision Res 12: 395

Pedler CMH, Tansley K (1963) The fine structure of the cone of a diurnal gecko (Phelsuma inunguis). Exp Eye Res 2: 39

Pennycuick CJ (1960) The physical basis of astronavigation in birds: Theoretical considerations. J Exp Biol 37: 573

Penrose LS, Penrose R (1958) Impossible objects: A special type of illusion. Br J Psychol 49: 31

Pettigrew JD (1972) The neurophysiology of binocular vision. Sci Am 227(2): 84

Pirenne MH (1967) Vision and the eye (2nd edition). Chapman & Hall, London, pp 224

Polyak S (1941) The retina. University of Chicago Press, Chicago

Polyak S (1968) The vertebrate visual system. University of Chicago Press, Chicago, London, pp 1390

Pothier F, Ali MA (1978) Étude du pigment scotopique chez trois Percidae: Perca flavescens, Stizostedion vitreum et S. canadense. Rev Can Biol 37: 91

Powers MK, Easter SS (1978) Absolute visual sensitivity of the goldfish. Vision Res 18: 1137

Pumphrey RJ (1948) The theory of the fovea. J Exp Biol 25: 299

Quaranta JV (1949) The color discrimination of Testudo vicina. Anat Rec 105: 510

Quaranta JV (1952) An experimental study of the color vision of the giant tortoise. Zoologica 37: 295

Reuter TE, White RH, Wald G (1971) Rhodopsin and porphyropsin fields in the adult bull frog retina. J Gen Physiol 58: 351

Riggs LA, Johnson EP, Schick AMI (1966) Electrical responses of the human eye to changes in wavelength of the stimulating light. J Opt Soc Am 56: 1621

Ripps H, Weale RA (1963) Cone pigments in the normal human fovea. Vision Res 3: 531

Rivamonte A (1976) Eye model to account for comparable aerial and underwater acuities of the bottlenose dolphin. Neth J Sea Res 10: 491

Rochon-Duvigneaud A (1943) Les yeux et la vision des vertébrés. Masson et Cie, Paris, pp 719

Romer AS, Grove BH (1935) Environment of the early vertebrates.

Rubin E (1915) Synoplevede Figurer. In: Beardslee DC, Wertheimer M (eds), Translation in readings in perception. Princeton, 1958

Samoiloff A, Pheophilaktova A (1907) Über die Farbenwahrnehmung beim Hunde. Zentralbl Physiol 21: 133

Sarnat HB, Netsky MG (1974) Visual system and dorsal thalamus. In: Evolution of the nervous system. Oxford University Press, New York, p 149

Schnetkamp PPM (1980) Ion selectivity of the cation transport system of isolated intact cattle rod outer segments: Evidence for a direct communication between the rod plasma membrane and the rod disk membrane. Biochim Biophys Acta 598: 66

Schultze M (1866) Zur Anatomie und Physiologie der Retina. Arch Mikroskop Anat 2: 165

Seliger HH (1977) Environmental photobiology. In: Smith KC (ed), The science of photobiology. Plenum, New York, p 143

Shapley R, Gordon J (1980) The visual sensitivity of the retina of the conger eel. Proc R Soc Lond 209B: 317

Shichi H (1971) Circular dichroism of bovine rhodopsin. Photochem Photobiol 13: 499

Shlaer R (1972) An eagle's eye: Quality of the retinal image. Science 176: 920

Sivak JG (1977) The role of the spectacle in the visual optics of the snake eye. Vision Res 17: 293

Sivak JG (1980) Accommodation in vertebrates: A contemporary survey. Curr Top Eye Res 3: 281

Sivak JG, Allen DB (1975) An evaluation of the 'ramp' retina of the horse. Vision Res 15: 1353

Sivak JG, Bobier WR, Levy B (1978) Refractive significance of nictitating membrane of bird eye. J Comp Physiol 125A: 335

Smith HW (1932) Water regulation and its evolution in the fishes. Quart Rev Biol 7: 1

Somiya H (1976) Functional significance of the yellow lens in the eyes of Argyropelecus affinis. Mar Biol 34: 93

Somiya H (1979) 'Yellow lens' eyes and luminous organs of Echiostoma barbatum (Stomiatoidei, Melanostomiatidae). Jpn J Ichthyol 25: 269

Somiya H (1980) Fishes with eye shine: Functional morphology of guanine tapetum lucidum. Mar Ecol Prog Ser 2: 9

Somiya H, Tamura T (1973) Studies on the visual accommodation in fishes. Jpn J Ichthyol 20: 193

Sorbi RT (1981) Modulation of sodium conductance in photo-receptor membranes by calcium ions and cGMP. Curr Top Memb Transp 15: 331

Spence KW (1934) Visual acuity and its relation to brightness in chimpanzee and man. J Comp Psychol 18: 333

Stell WK (1967) The structure and relationships of horizontal cells and photoreceptor bipolar synaptic complexes in goldfish retina. Am J Anat 120: 401

Stewart VM (1971) A cross-cultural test of the "Carpentered Environment" hypothesis using three geometric illusions in Zambia. Doctoral Dissertation, University of Illinois, Urbana, Illinois

Stryer L, Hurley JB, Fung BKK (1981) First stage amplification in the cyclic-nucleotide cascade of vision. Curr Top Memb Transp 15: 93

Studnicka FK (1898) Untersuchungen über den Bau der Sehnerven der Wirbeltiere. Jena Zeits f Naturwiss 31: 1

Symthe RH (1975) Vision in the animal world. MacMillan Press Ltd, London, pp 165

Szuts EZ (1981) Calcium tracer exchange in the rods of excised retinas. Curr Top Memb Transp 15: 291

Szuts EZ, Cone RA (1977) Calcium content of frog rod outer segments and discs. Biochim Biophys Acta 468: 194

Tansley K (1931) The regeneration of visual purple with special reference to dark adaptation and night blindness. J Physiol 71: 442

Tansley K (1959) The retina of two nocturnal geckos, Hemidactylus turcicus and Tarentola mauritanica. Pflüger's Arch 26: 213

Tansley K (1965) Vision in vertebrates. Chapman & Hall, London, pp 132

Taylor DH, Adler K (1978) The pineal body: Site of extraocular perception of celestial cues for orientation in tiger salaman-der (Ambystoma tigrinum). J Comp Physiol 124: 357

Tigges J (1963) Untersuchungen über den Farbensinn von Tupaia glis (Diard 1820). Z Morphol Anthropol 53: 109

Tokuyasu K, Yamada E (1959) The fine structure of the retina studied with electron microscope. IV. Morphogenesis of outer segments of retinal rods. J Biophys Biochem Cytol 6: 225

Tokuyasu K, Yamada E (1960) The fine structure of the retina. V. Abnormal retinal rods and their morphogenesis. J Biophys Biochem Cytol 7: 187

Tomita T (1950) Studies on the intraretinal action potential. Part I. Relation between localization of micropipette in the retina and the shape of the intraretinal action potential. Jpn J Physiol 1: 110

Tsin ATC, Beatty DD (1977) Visual pigment changes in rainbow trout in response to temperature. Science 195: 1385

Vakkur GJ, Bishop PO (1963) The schematic eye of the cat. Vision Res 3: 357

Valentin G (1879a) Ein beitrag zur Kenntnis der Brechungsverhältnisse der Thiergewebe. Pflüger's Arch 19: 78

Valentin G (1879b) Fortgesetzte Untersuchungen über die Brechungsverhältnisse der Thiergewebe. Pflüger's Arch 20: 283

van Veen T, Hartwig HG, Müller K (1976) Light-dependent motor activity and photonegative behavior in the eel (Anguilla anguilla L.). Evidence for extraretinal and extrapineal photoreception. J Comp Physiol 111: 209

Wagner HJ (1978) Cell types and connectivity patterns in mosaic retinas. Adv Anat Embryol Cell Biol, vol 55. Springer-Verlag, Heidelberg, pp 81

Wagner HJ, Ali MA (1978) Retinal organisation in goldeye and mooneye (Teleostei: Hiodontidae). Rev Can Biol 37: 65

Wagner HJ, Menezes NA, Ali MA (1976) Retinal adaptations in some Brazilian tide pool fishes (Teleostei). Zoomorph 83: 209

Wald G (1935) Carotenoids and the visual cycle. J Gen Physiol 19: 351

Wald G (1939) The porphyropsin visual system. J Gen Physiol 22: 775

Wald G (1942) The visual system and vitamins A of the sea lamprey. J Gen Physiol 25: 331

Wald G (1964) The receptors of human color vision. Science 145: 1007

Walls GL (1937) Significance of the foveal depression. Arch Ophthalmol NY 18: 912

Walls GL (1940) Ophthalmological implications for the early history of the snakes. Copeia 1

Walls GL (1942) The vertebrate eye and its adaptive radiation. Cranbrook Inst Sci, Bloomfield Hills, Michigan, pp 785

Warren RH, Burnside B (1978) Microtubules in cone myoid elongation in the teleost retina. J Cell Biol 78: 247

Weale RA (1965) Vision and fundus reflectometry: A review.

Photochem Photobiol 4: 67

Weale RA (1968) Photochemistry of the human central fovea. Nature 218: 238

Wiesel TN, Hubel DH (1966) Spatial and chromatic interactions in the lateral geniculate body of the rhesus monkey. J Neurophysiol 29: 1115

Woodruff ML, Bownds MD (1979) Amplitude, kinetics and reversibility of a light-induced decrease in guanosine 3',5'-cyclic monophosphate in frog photoreceptor membranes. J Gen Physiol 73: 629

Wurtman RJ (1975) The effects of light on man and other mammals. Ann Rev Physiol 37: 467

Wyszecki G, Stiles WS (1967) Colour science. Wiley & Sons Inc, New York

Yau KW, McNaughton PA, Hodgkin AL (1981) Effects of ions on the light-sensitive current in retinal rods. Nature 292: 502

Yokoyama K, Oksche A, Darden ThR, Farner DS (1978) The sites of encephalic photoreception in photoperiod induction of the growth of the testes in the white-crowned sparrow, Zonotrichia leucophys gambellî. Cell Tissue Res 189: 441

Yoshikami S, Hagins WA (1971) Light, calcium and the photocurrent of rods and cones. Biophys J 11: 47

Young T (1802) On the theory of light and colours. Phil Trans R Soc. Part 1, 20. Reprinted in Lectures on natural philosophy, 1 st ed, vol 2. London, 1807, p 613

Zorn M, Futterman S (1971) Properties of rhodopsin dependent on associated phospholipid. J Biol Chem 246: 881

Zweig M, Snyder SH, Axelrod J (1966) Evidence for a nonretinal pathway of light to the pineal gland of new born rats. Proc Natl Acad Sci USA 56: 515

Zyznar ES, Larson WL, Ali MA (1978) Microspectrophotometric studies on the visual pigment in the intact retina of the goldfish, Carassius auratus Linn. Rev Can Biol 37: 143

SYSTEMATIC INDEX

257

SUBJECT INDEX

Pages underlined refer to the figures and tables